Sports
Injuries

Diseases and Disorders

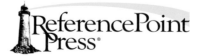

ReferencePoint
Press®

San Diego, CA

Other books in the Compact Research Diseases and Disorders set:

ADHD
Anxiety Disorders
Bipolar Disorders
Drug Addiction
Food-Borne Illnesses
Herpes
HPV
Learning Disabilities
Mood Disorders
Obsessive-Compulsive Disorders
Personality Disorders
Post-Traumatic Stress Disorders
Self-Injury Disorders
Sexually Transmitted Diseases

*For a complete list of titles please visit www.referencepointpress.com.

Sports Injuries

Peggy J. Parks

Diseases and Disorders

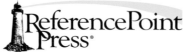

ReferencePoint
Press®

San Diego, CA

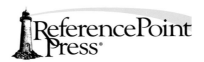
ReferencePoint Press®

© 2013 ReferencePoint Press, Inc.
Printed in the United States

For more information, contact:
ReferencePoint Press, Inc.
PO Box 27779
San Diego, CA 92198
www.ReferencePointPress.com

Picture credits:
Cover: Dreamstime and iStockphoto.com
Maury Aaseng: 33–35, 47–49, 61–62, 75–77
AP Images: 12
Du Cane Medical Imaging LTD/Science Photo Library: 14

LIBRARY OF CONGRESS CATALOGING-IN-PUBLICATION DATA

Parks, Peggy J., 1951–
   Sports injuries / by Peggy J. Parks.
     p. cm. -- (Compact research series)
   Includes bibliographical references and index.
   ISBN-13: 978-1-60152-244-3 (hardback)
   ISBN-10: 1-60152-244-4 (hardback)
  1. Sports injuries. I. Title.
   RD97.P37   2011
   617.1'027--dc23
                                                     2011041355

Contents

Foreword

"Where is the knowledge we have lost in information?"

—T.S. Eliot, "The Rock."

As modern civilization continues to evolve, its ability to create, store, distribute, and access information expands exponentially. The explosion of information from all media continues to increase at a phenomenal rate. By 2020 some experts predict the worldwide information base will double every 73 days. While access to diverse sources of information and perspectives is paramount to any democratic society, information alone cannot help people gain knowledge and understanding. Information must be organized and presented clearly and succinctly in order to be understood. The challenge in the digital age becomes not the creation of information, but how best to sort, organize, enhance, and present information.

ReferencePoint Press developed the *Compact Research* series with this challenge of the information age in mind. More than any other subject area today, researching current issues can yield vast, diverse, and unqualified information that can be intimidating and overwhelming for even the most advanced and motivated researcher. The *Compact Research* series offers a compact, relevant, intelligent, and conveniently organized collection of information covering a variety of current topics ranging from illegal immigration and deforestation to diseases such as anorexia and meningitis.

The series focuses on three types of information: objective single-author narratives, opinion-based primary source quotations, and facts

and statistics. The clearly written objective narratives provide context and reliable background information. Primary source quotes are carefully selected and cited, exposing the reader to differing points of view, and facts and statistics sections aid the reader in evaluating perspectives. Presenting these key types of information creates a richer, more balanced learning experience.

For better understanding and convenience, the series enhances information by organizing it into narrower topics and adding design features that make it easy for a reader to identify desired content. For example, in *Compact Research: Illegal Immigration*, a chapter covering the economic impact of illegal immigration has an objective narrative explaining the various ways the economy is impacted, a balanced section of numerous primary source quotes on the topic, followed by facts and full-color illustrations to encourage evaluation of contrasting perspectives.

The ancient Roman philosopher Lucius Annaeus Seneca wrote, "It is quality rather than quantity that matters." More than just a collection of content, the *Compact Research* series is simply committed to creating, finding, organizing, and presenting the most relevant and appropriate amount of information on a current topic in a user-friendly style that invites, intrigues, and fosters understanding.

Sports Injuries at a Glance

Types of Sports Injuries

The two types of sports injuries are acute and chronic. Acute injuries happen suddenly, such as sprains or broken bones, whereas chronic injuries develop over time.

Most Common Sports Injuries

According to the National Institute of Arthritis and Musculoskeletal and Skin Diseases (NIAMS), sprains and strains are among the most common sports injuries, as are injuries to the knee, swollen muscles, and fractures.

Concussions

A concussion is a traumatic brain injury, and typical symptoms include headaches, blurred vision, dizziness, and memory loss. The athlete may lose consciousness, but this does not happen with most concussions.

Concussion Danger

An athlete who has sustained a concussion is four to six times more likely to sustain a second concussion if another head injury occurs. This can lead to a deadly condition called second-impact syndrome.

Prevalence of Sports Injuries

According to the Centers for Disease Control and Prevention (CDC), sports- and recreation-related injuries affect about 7 million people each year in the United States.

Seriousness of Youth Sports Injuries

The CDC states that of the estimated 7 million sports injuries that occur each year, over half are among children and adolescents.

Treatment

Treatments vary, with some injuries requiring only rest, ice, compression, and elevation, and other injuries requiring major surgery.

Sports Injury Prevention

Experts say that better protective gear (including helmets), improved physical fitness, and tougher rules, such as those that apply to potential head injuries, can all help prevent sport injuries.

Overview

Nathan Stiles had everything going for him. The 17-year-old from Spring Hill, Kansas, was a 4.0 student, homecoming king, and a star athlete on his high school basketball and football teams. Often called "Superman" by his teammates, Stiles was a true competitor who refused to quit even when he was injured. So in early October 2010, when he started to complain about headaches, it was totally out of character for him. The football season was under way, and Stiles had been hit hard in a couple of games. His coaches sidelined him and his mother took him to a medical center, where he underwent a series of tests, including a computerized axial tomography scan. Although the tests found nothing wrong, doctors suspected that Stiles had a concussion and advised him not to play football until the headaches went away. A few weeks later he assured his parents that his head no longer hurt and he felt good enough to get back in the game.

On October 28, 2010, Stiles played in the last football game of the season. During one pass interception he hit the ground hard, and soon afterward he stumbled off the field, screaming that his head hurt. He then collapsed unconscious on the ground and was transported by helicopter to the hospital, where a team of doctors performed emergency surgery. They could not save him, however, as Stiles's brain was bleeding and severely swollen. He died the next morning. An autopsy determined that the cause of death was a "rebleed" of a subdural hematoma, or the pooling of blood on the brain's surface that had not been detected in earlier tests. His grief-stricken parents could not help wondering if he had been hiding his pain from them so he could keep playing football. "Even if he was," says his mother, "what kid thinks, 'Oh, I'm going to die from a headache?' He's a 17-year-old kid. They don't think they're going to die from anything."[1]

Dangerous Sports

Hard hitting is as much a part of football as running and passing. Because of the head injuries that can result from those hits, football is considered one of the most dangerous sports, as *Time* sports journalist Sean Gregory writes: "Football has been a rough sport since the leather-helmet days, but today's version raises the violence to an art form."[2] According to the American Association of Neurological Surgeons, the incidence of football-related concussion in the United States is estimated at 300,000 per year. Because many concussions are never diagnosed and/or reported, experts say that the actual number is likely much higher.

Some Olympic sports are also dangerous, and experts say they are becoming more so. A notable example is snowboarding, in which athletes perform flips and spins high in the air before landing on a trough-shaped surface known as a half-pipe. Such stunts are very familiar to world-champion snowboarder Kevin Pearce—and one

> " Hard hitting is as much a part of football as running and passing. Because of the head injuries that can result from those hits, football is considered one of the most dangerous sports. "

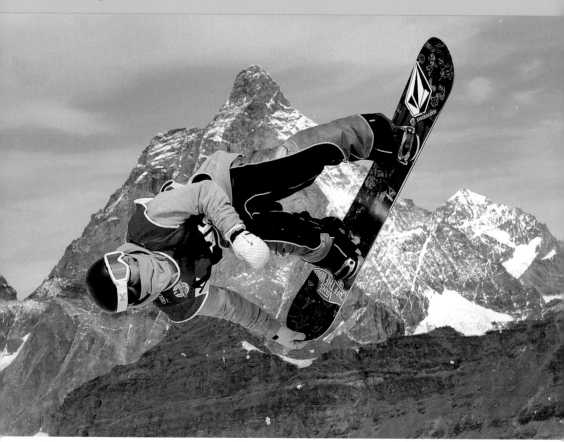

Hard-hitting contact sports such as football and sports that involve high-flying flips and spins such as snowboarding (pictured), often lead to injuries. Sprains, strains, and fractures are among the most common injuries in various sports but concussions represent a growing concern.

he performed in December 2009 nearly cost him his life. Pearce was training in Park City, Utah, for the upcoming Winter Olympic Games. While performing a twisting back flip known as a double cork, he attempted to land and slammed the right side of his head against the hard, icy surface of the half-pipe.

The blow caused such severe damage to Pearce's brain that doctors were not sure if he would survive. He did, but for three agonizing months he underwent eight hours of rehabilitation every day as he relearned how to walk, talk, and take care of himself. Within a year he had made amazing progress, able to play golf and tennis and anticipating the day that doctors clear him to snowboard again. But even when they do, Pearce

knows that his days as an Olympic competitor are over, and that is tough for him. Standing at the foot of a mountain in Aspen, Colorado, during January 2011, he said to a reporter: "There's nothing I would rather do than ride this pipe right now. You don't realize what it is till you lose it."[3]

What Are Sports Injuries?

Sports injuries are loosely divided into two categories: acute and chronic. Acute sports injuries are those that happen suddenly, such as when an athlete breaks (or fractures) a bone or sustains a sprain or strain. The latter two terms are sometimes used interchangeably, but they are not the same. A sprain occurs when an athlete stretches or tears ligaments, which are tissues that connect bones together at a joint. Strains also involve stretches or tears, but they affect muscles or tendons, the fibrous tissues that attach muscle to bone.

Unlike the suddenness of acute injuries, those of the chronic type develop over a period of time. Most common are overuse injuries, as orthopedic (sometimes spelled *orthopaedic*) surgeon Joseph Iero explains: "All active persons, from the elite athlete to the 'weekend warrior,' are subject to these injuries that typically become chronic because they do not cause enough discomfort to cause the athlete to stop participating in their sport."[4] One example of an overuse injury is tennis elbow, in which tendons on the outside of the forearm become overworked and inflamed.

Another type of chronic injury is the stress fracture, which begins as a tiny crack in a bone. These fractures typically develop in the feet and legs and are most common among athletes who participate in running/jumping sports that involve repetitive impact, such as gymnastics or track and field. A world-champion gymnast who sustained a stress fracture is 18-year-old Rebecca Bross. In December 2010 she underwent surgery, in which doctors inserted two screws into her ankle bone to ensure that the fracture healed properly.

> " Anyone who participates in sports is at risk of getting hurt at some point, but the more aggressive the sport, the greater the risk of injury. "

Common Sports Injuries

Anyone who participates in sports is at risk of getting hurt at some point, but the more aggressive the sport, the greater the risk of injury. According to the NIAMS, common sports-related injuries include sprains and

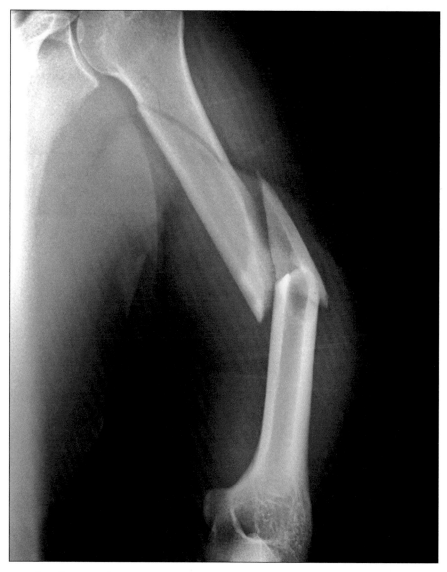

A colored X-ray shows multiple fractures in a patient's upper arm bone. In some cases, once broken bones are set they can heal on their own, but more severe breaks often require surgery. No matter which form of treatment is needed, full recovery takes time.

strains, injuries to the knee, swollen muscles, and fractures. Dislocations, which result from two bones that form a joint becoming separated, are more common in some sports than others, as the NIAMS reports: "Contact sports such as football and basketball, as well as high-impact sports and sports that can result in excessive stretching or falling, cause the majority of dislocations."[5]

Neck injuries happen most often to athletes who partici-pate in sports such as football, rugby, horseback riding, gym-nastics, and water sports. Especially common is an injury known as a stinger (or burner), in which nerves in the neck are stretched. Florida Hospital Sports Medicine explains: "In contact or collision sports, burn-ers and stingers are very common injuries. The injury is named for the stinging or burning pain that spreads from the shoulder to the hand. It is often described as feeling like an electric shock or lightning bolt shooting down the arm, often with a warm sensation accompanying it."[6]

> " One of the challenges of diagnosing con-cussions is that they cannot be detected in tests such as mag-netic resonance imaging (MRI) and computed tomog-raphy (CT) scans, unless there is obvi-ous bleeding and/or brain swelling. "

The Danger of Concussions

The word *concussion* is taken from the Latin verb *concutere*, meaning "to shake violently," which is a fitting description of this brain injury. The soft, gelatin-like brain is encased within the hard, bony skull. It floats in cerebrospinal fluid, which acts as a liquid cushion to protect it against normal bumps and movements. But when someone sustains a hard blow to the head, this causes the brain to bang into the skull. The CDC explains: "This sudden movement of the brain can cause the brain to bounce around or twist in the skull, stretching and damaging the brain cells and creating chemical changes in the brain. These chemical changes can lead to short- or long-term problems with thinking, learning, lan-guage, and emotions, until the brain recovers."[7]

When an athlete has sustained a concussion, he or she often feels mentally foggy and has trouble remembering recent events, and may also suffer from headaches and sensitivity to bright lights and loud noises. But concussions are challenging to diagnose because they cannot be detected on magnetic resonance imaging (MRI) or computerized tomography (CT) scans unless there are physical changes in the brain, such as bleeding or swelling. As a result, physicians can only make concussion diagnoses based on an athlete's symptoms.

> A study published in September 2010 in the medical journal *Pediatrics* showed that 375,000 children and teenagers are treated in hospital emergency rooms each year for basketball-related injuries.

One of the greatest risks of concussions is that they can lead to devastating long-term brain damage. Over the course of his career as a professional hockey player, Eric Lindros sustained at least eight concussions. He retired in 2007 and has only recently spoken publicly about the effects these brain injuries have had on him. His personality changed, and he became depressed and developed a paralyzing fear of public speaking or being in a crowd. He explains why he hid these factors from everyone—even from himself—for a very long time: "You got to understand, you want to wake up in the morning and you want to look at yourself and say, 'I've got the perfect engine to accomplish what I need to in this game tonight.' You are not going to look in the mirror and say, 'Boy, I'm depressed.'"[8]

Prevalence of Sports Injuries

According to the CDC, each year approximately 7 million sports- and recreation-related injuries occur in the United States, and statistics about these injuries are typically compiled separately for each sport. According to the American Academy of Orthopaedic Surgeons, for example, over 63,000 hockey-related injuries are treated in US hospitals, doctors' offices, clinics, outpatient surgery centers, and emergency rooms each year. A 2010 report based on data from the US Consumer Product Safety

Commission showed that 446,788 sports-related head injuries were treated at American hospital emergency rooms in 2009, which was an increase of nearly 95,000 over 2008.

A report in the September 2010 issue of the *British Journal of Sports Medicine* showed that 11 percent of athletes sustained injuries during the 2010 Winter Olympics. The incidence, however, differed among the various sports, with up to 35 percent of athletes in bobsled, ice hockey, alpine freestyle skiing, snowboarding, and skeleton events being injured. The most common injuries were bruising, as well as sprains and strains. Many of the athletes were injured during practice runs before the actual competitions began—including one who tragically died. Nodar Kumari-tashvili, a 21-year-old luger from the former Soviet republic of Georgia, was killed when his sled crashed during a practice run. According to Olympics historian David Wallechinsky, this was the first competition-related death in the history of the Winter Olympic Games.

Sports Injury Warning Signs

When an athlete has been injured, the symptoms depend on the type and severity of the injury. Sprains, for example, typically result in tenderness and/or pain, bruising, and swelling. Strains tend to be accompanied by muscle spasms and loss of strength, whereas fractures involve pain that worsens as weight is put on the broken bone. If a fracture is severe, an athlete can experience excruciating pain—as Buster Posey learned on May 26, 2011. Posey is a catcher for the San Francisco Giants baseball team. During a game against the Florida Marlins, he was attempting to block home plate when a Marlins player running in from third base crashed into him. Afterward, Posey lay on the ground, writhing in pain. X-rays later showed that he had fractured his lower left leg and would not be able to play baseball for the rest of the season.

Pain is also a factor for many who injure the Achilles tendon, which is a strong, rope-like cord that connects the calf muscle to the heel bone. Injuries result from the tendon being stretched or torn and most commonly affect athletes in sports that involve running and/or jumping. The symptoms of an Achilles tendon injury vary widely, from a sensation of being kicked in the back of the leg, with little or no pain resulting, to pain so severe that it seems unbearable. According to the NIAMS, Achilles tendon injuries are some of the most painful of all sports injuries, as

the agency explains: "These injuries can be so sudden and agonizing that they have been known to bring down charging professional football players in shocking fashion."[9]

How Serious a Problem Are Injuries in Youth Sports?

According to the NIAMS, each year over 38 million children and adolescents participate in organized sports in the United States (such as on school teams or community leagues), with still more involved in recreational sports. The benefits are immense, from keeping kids in shape to learning the value of working hard to achieve personal goals. But the downside of sports involvement is that young people may be injured—and according to an April 2011 report by Safe Kids USA, sports-related injuries among youth are on the rise. The proportion of young athletes who were injured during team sports has increased 3 percent over the past decade, with an even bigger spike among youth who had multiple injuries. The study found that the rate of multiple injuries in team sports increased from 15 percent in January 2000 to 21 percent in March 2011.

> In order to relieve pain and reduce swelling, sports medicine specialists commonly recommend RICE, which is an acronym for *rest, ice, compression,* and *elevation.*

Of all the sports that involve young males, studies consistently show that football is the riskiest. Another high-risk sport, for girls as well as boys, is basketball. An 11-year study published in September 2010 in the medical journal *Pediatrics* showed that 375,000 children and teenagers were treated in hospital emergency rooms each year for basketball-related injuries. In examining gender differences, the researchers found that boys were most likely to suffer from cuts, fractures, and dislocations, while girls most often sustained head or knee injuries. A particularly disturbing finding was that the number of basketball-related concussions among youth rose 70 percent between 1997 and 2007, with the largest increase among girls.

How Are Sports Injuries Treated?

Because of the differences among various sports-related injuries, recommended treatments vary. Initially, many injuries can be treated at home without a doctor's care. In order to relieve pain and reduce swelling, sports medicine specialists commonly recommend RICE, which stands for *rest, ice, compression,* and *elevation.* For a sprained ankle, for instance, a patient would be advised to avoid putting weight on it, to apply an ice pack to the sprain for 20 minutes up to eight times a day, to wrap the ankle with an elastic bandage, and if possible, to keep the ankle elevated on a pillow to help control swelling. If pain continues and/or swelling gets worse, the patient will be advised to seek medical attention.

In some cases surgery may be required, for example, to repair torn connective tissue or to realign bones after a serious fracture. When Ryan O'Keefe was a senior in high school, he sustained an injury that required surgery. O'Keefe was a linebacker for his school football team in Grovetown, Georgia. In the final game of the season, he was hit in the head by an opposing player and immediately felt tingling and numbness in his neck. This is a typical symptom of a stinger, but when the pain did not go away, O'Keefe had X-rays and learned that he had fractured a vertebra in his neck. He underwent surgery, during which doctors removed a disc between two of his vertebrae, inserted a metal plate in its place, and stabilized it with screws.

The Long Road Back

Serious sports injuries often require rehabilitation to help athletes regain physical function, with the initial goal of getting pain and inflammation under control. Graduated exercise plays an important role in this process, as Daniel Evans, a physical therapist from Plano, Texas, explains:

> Once you've reduced the swelling, you want the patient to be able to return to normal range of motion or mobility. You want to start restoring the available range, progressing slowly. The balance, or art, of rehabilitation is to get the patient back to maximum range of motion without inflaming or bringing back the pain. You are constantly trying to balance that through rehabilitation.[10]

> **For some athletes, rehabilitation after an injury is a long, difficult, and painful process.**

Yet for some athletes, rehabilitation after an injury is a long, difficult, and painful process. No one knows this better than Denise Castelli, who broke her leg in 2008 while sliding into a base during a softball game. Before long she developed complications, including a severe infection, and had to have her leg amputated below the knee. Once Castelli was physically ready, she went through four months of grueling physical therapy while she learned how to walk on her artificial leg—and her recovery was remarkable. Not only did she return to playing softball, she was also selected to be a ball girl during the US Open Tennis Championships in September 2011.

How Can Sports Injuries Be Prevented?

Health experts emphasize that many—and perhaps even most—sports injuries are preventable. According to sports medicine specialist Tim Greene, the most common cause is inadequate preparation, which leads to overuse of joints or muscles. This could be avoided through better physical conditioning, as he explains:

> Many sports-related injuries can be traced to a lack of core body strength—which is the strength of the muscles of the torso that keep your stomach strong and support your back. Think of the body as a tree that has strong branches but a weak trunk. That imbalance of strength can cause strain, cracking and even collapse the trunk. If your core is not strong and you engage in a running or jumping activity, your risk for injury is increased.[11]

A major preventive measure for many sports is protective equipment. This is especially true for high-contact sports that carry a high risk of head injury, which leads most experts to agree that properly designed helmets are essential. But physicians who specialize in sports injuries make it clear that helmets cannot necessarily prevent concussions, so the emphasis must be on stopping athletes from intentionally hitting each other

head-on. Robert C. Cantu, a Boston neurosurgeon and noted expert on sports-related concussions, states: "The No. 1 thing: take the purposeful helmet hit out of football, for both blocking and tackling . . . you don't need all this one-on-one helmet-on-helmet macho stuff."[12]

Injuries Are a Part of Sports

Millions of people of all ages play sports and enjoy the benefits of doing so. Unfortunately, though, sports participation and injuries often go hand in hand. The majority of sports injuries are mild, involving bruises or sprains that heal over a short period of time, but some are serious enough to be life-threatening. With greater awareness of sports injuries, along with measures put into place that can help prevent them, perhaps fewer athletes will end up getting hurt while doing what they love.

What Are Sports Injuries?

66Sports and injuries go hand in hand. With the brutal beating that the body takes from countless training reps and the rigors of hard-core performance on the field, injuries will happen. And there are certain parts of the body that remain the most prone to injury.99

—Rick Lehman, a physician and medical director of the US Center for Sports Medicine.

66Regardless of type, physical activity and sports participation carry some risk of injury, whether it's working up a blister while walking in new shoes, pulling a leg muscle while cycling, or jamming a finger in a volleyball game.99

—Gordon Edlin and Eric Golanty, college professors from California and coauthors of the book *Health & Wellness*.

Each year during late summer, hundreds of cyclists converge on upstate New York's Catskill Mountains for the Tour of the Catskills race. University of Pennsylvania junior Colby Samstag participated in the August 2011 race, along with fellow members of the Penn Cycling Club. On the first day Samstag came in seventy-ninth, rising to sixty-third place the next day. On the third day of the race things were looking good for Samstag, as he led a pack of cyclists downhill, speeding along at approximately 50 miles per hour (80.5kph). Then, seemingly out of nowhere, a sport-utility vehicle appeared on the road in front of the cyclists and abruptly stopped. With no way to avoid a collision, Samstag smashed into the SUV and flew head-first through its windshield.

Samstag was critically injured in the crash. He sustained neck and head injuries, including to his eye socket, jaw, and ear, as well as fractured bones in his elbow and hand. Hundreds of stitches were necessary to repair numerous cuts along his jaw, neck, arm, hip, and fingers. After a few days in the hospital, Samstag was able to get up and walk, although he was still suffering from neck pain. In an interview several weeks after the crash, he said that he was getting better each day, but he knew that the recovery process would be long and might keep him from accomplishing a personal goal. "I had dreams of being a pro cyclist someday," says Samstag, "but I don't know if it'll happen."[13]

Eyesight at Risk

Fortunately for Samstag, the eye socket injury he sustained did not permanently harm his vision—but after smashing through a glass windshield, he could easily have been blinded. Eye injuries are among the most serious risks for athletes. According to the National Eye Institute, over 100,000 sports-related eye injuries occur each year in the United States, and nearly half require a visit to hospital emergency departments. The severity of sports-related eye injuries can vary from mild scrapes of the cornea (the clear, dome-shaped surface at the front of the eye) to blunt trauma caused by an object directly hitting the eye.

Ice hockey players who do not wear protective face shields have an extremely high risk of sustaining eye injuries because they can get hit in the face with another player's stick. Even more dangerous is being hit with a hockey puck—which streaks through the air at about 100 miles per hour (161kph). That is what happened to Manny Malhotra, a player for the Canadian pro hockey team Vancouver Canucks. During a game on March 16, 2011, a puck deflected off a player's stick and smacked Malhotra in the left eye. The injury nearly cost him his eyesight

> " Ice hockey players who do not wear protective face shields have an extremely high risk of sustaining eye injuries because they can get hit in the face with another player's stick. "

and his career. But after two surgeries, doctors were able to save Malhotra's eyesight. Less than three months after he was injured, he returned to the ice for the Stanley Cup playoffs—but this time he was wearing a full-face Plexiglas shield.

Luis Salazar was also hit in the left eye, with a baseball rather than a hockey puck—but his story did not end as happily as Malhotra's. Salazar is a manager for the Atlanta Braves' minor league team and a former pro baseball player. On March 9, 2011, during a spring training game in Kissimmee, Florida, he was standing on the top step of a dugout when a speeding foul ball slammed into his face and knocked him unconscious. He was airlifted to a hospital in Orlando, where he was treated for multiple facial fractures. Doctors were unable to save his eye, and it was surgically removed on March 15. Two weeks later Salazar returned to training camp, and despite losing his eye, he was feeling positive. "I'm very fortunate to be alive," he says. "God gave me a second chance in this life, and I'm going to take advantage of it."[14]

> " Sports medicine specialists and health organizations say that overuse is the most common cause of sports injuries. "

Overused and Damaged

Sports medicine specialists and health organizations say that overuse is the most common cause of sports injuries. According to physical therapist Robert Donatelli, overuse injuries are difficult to diagnose because of their gradual onset and pain that comes and goes. He says overuse injuries are often caused by muscle dysfunction. "If some muscles fatigue because of prolonged activities such as tennis," he says, "the muscle is no longer an effective shock absorber. As a result of fatigue the muscle can become damaged, resulting in weakness, poor flexibility, and inadequate endurance."[15] Donatelli adds that the knee is highly susceptible to overuse injuries because of muscle imbalance. For instance, weakness in the hamstrings (the three muscles that run down the back of the thigh) can increase strain on the anterior cruciate ligament (ACL). One of four ligaments in the knee joint that connect the shinbone to the thighbone, the

ACL is critical to knee stability. An athlete who sustains an ACL injury often feels a pop in the knee, similar to the snapping of a rubber band, followed by the knee buckling or shifting.

An ACL injury ended Laura DeBruler's reign as a college volleyball star. For eight years she dominated the court, first with her high school in Downers Grove, Illinois, and then with the University of Illinois. DeBruler was ranked among the best in the United States, but her starring role on the college team came to an abrupt end on October 12, 2010, during a match against the University of Michigan. She explains: "I went for a ball that was very tight [to the net] and when I came down . . . my left leg took all the weight and that's when my knee went out. I was devastated, especially with it being senior year and we had so many big plans to do great things. It was something that you never think it will happen to you until it happens."[16]

On November 17, 2010, DeBruler had surgery to repair her injured ACL, and then went through months of rehabilitation. While she was sidelined she continued to root for her teammates, traveling with them to volleyball matches and acting as an assistant coach. "Since I couldn't play," she says, "I had to take on more of a vocal role and be a cheerleader. I never expected to be that type of person for the team. Now I've embraced it my senior year."[17] Despite the setback of her injury, DeBruler still dreams of a future that involves volleyball. She hopes to play on a professional team in Europe. "I want to play as long as I can," she says, "and then if my body can't take it or I don't like it any more, I'll come home and coach here."[18]

> " When pain is the only symptom, many athletes keep playing no matter how bad they are hurting— and this can lead to serious long-term problems. "

Playing Through Pain

ACL injuries cannot be ignored, because the knees give out and the athlete has a hard time standing up. But when pain is the only symptom, many athletes keep playing no matter how bad they are hurting. Says Marjorie J. Albohm, who is president of the National Athletic Trainers'

Association: "We have been fighting the 'playing through pain' culture since as long as we've been in existence, since 1950, when the organization was founded."[19]

Alpine ski racer Lindsey Vonn understands playing through pain. A week before the 2010 Winter Olympics, she was practicing in Austria when she severely twisted her right leg. She then tumbled over the top of her skis and smashed her shin against the top of her boot. Vonn had a deep muscle bruise that caused her terrible pain, as she explained a short time after the accident: "When I tried my boot on, I was just standing there in the hotel room barely flexing forward, and it was excruciatingly painful. And I've got to try to ski downhill at 75, 80 miles an hour with a lot of forces pushed up against my shin."[20] Vonn did ski. Two weeks after she was injured, she won the gold in the opening women's race and made Olympic history by being the first American woman to clinch a gold medal for downhill racing. In this instance, playing through pain worked out. It does not always happen that way. Some injuries just get worse and bring more pain.

Devastating Brain Trauma

Concussions are among the most dangerous sports injuries. Signs of concussion include headache, blurred vision, feeling dazed and confused, and memory problems, although symptoms vary based on the severity of damage to the brain. As the American Association of Neurological Surgeons writes: "Mild cases may result in a brief change in mental state or consciousness, while severe cases may result in extended periods of unconsciousness, coma, or even death."[21]

Once an athlete has sustained a concussion, he or she is four to six times more likely to suffer a second concussion in the event of another head injury. This can lead to grave consequences as Terry Zeigler, a certified athletic trainer who specializes in the prevention, treatment, and rehabilitation of injuries, explains: "Because the brain is more vulnerable and susceptible to injury after an initial brain injury, it only takes a minimal force to cause irreversible damage."[22] Sustaining a second concussion can lead to a dangerous condition known as second-impact syndrome, whereby the brain swells rapidly and the brain stem shuts down. This often leads to death, as was the case with Nathan Stiles. If the athlete survives, he or she may suffer from catastrophic brain damage.

Zackery Lystedt was stricken with second-impact syndrome when he was in the eighth grade, and his life has never been the same. Lystedt was a linebacker on the football team at Tahoma Junior High School in Maple Valley, Washington. During a game on October 12, 2006, he smacked his head while tackling a running back, and afterward he lay on the ground, conscious but unable to get up. His coaches took him out for the final three plays of the second quarter, but then sent him back in the game after halftime. Lystedt made a tackle that helped clinch his team's win, and he was swarmed by team-mates—but then disaster struck. CBS Sports reporter Matt Rybaltowski writes: "Less than a minute later, after the teams exchanged handshakes, Lystedt turned to his father Victor and said, 'Dad, my head hurts.' Then, 'Dad, I can't see.' As his brain swelled severely and his optic nerve became impinged, Lystedt let out a blood-curdling scream and collapsed."[23]

> " Once an athlete has sustained a concussion, he or she is four to six times more likely to suffer a second concussion in the event of another head injury. "

Lystedt was airlifted to a hospital in Seattle, where doctors performed emergency surgery on his brain. Although they were able to save his life, he suffered severe brain damage that caused him to have numerous strokes and to spend three months in a coma. When he finally regained consciousness, he was paralyzed and could not speak or swallow. Lystedt began intensive physical therapy, and that, combined with his own fierce determination and hard work, helped him make amazing progress. Although he could not walk, he returned to school in a wheelchair, and in October 2010 his classmates elected him homecoming king. The following June, assisted by his best friend and inspired by a rousing standing ovation, Lystedt rose from his wheelchair and slowly walked across the stage to receive his high school diploma. "Words can't express how far I've come,"[24] he says.

Nothing to Take Lightly

Sports participation can result in a multitude of different injuries, from cuts and bruises to catastrophic damage to the brain. People who ride in

cycling races can get injured, as can those who skate, ski, play baseball, or make the winning play in a football game. Some insist that getting hurt is just part of being involved in sports, and to some extent that may be true. But if athletes value their health—and their lives—they must learn to be as cautious as possible, protect themselves, and pay close attention when their bodies signal that something is wrong.

What Are Sports Injuries?

66 Over the past several years, there has been growing and convincing evidence that repetitive concussive and subconcussive blows to the head in NFL players lead to a progressive neurodegenerative brain disease called chronic traumatic encephalopathy or CTE. 99

—Robert C. Cantu, testimony to the US House Judiciary Committee, October 28, 2009. http://judiciary.house.gov.

Cantu is a Boston neurosurgeon and cofounder of the Sports Legacy Institute and the Center for the Study of Traumatic Encephalopathy at Boston University School of Medicine.

66 There is not enough valid, reliable or objective scientific evidence at present to determine whether or not repeat head impacts in professional football result in long term brain damage. 99

—Ira Casson, testimony to the US House Judiciary Committee, January 4, 2010. http://judiciary.house.gov.

Casson is a neurologist from New York and former cochair of the NFL's panel on head injuries.

Bracketed quotes indicate conflicting positions.

* Editor's Note: While the definition of a primary source can be narrowly or broadly defined, for the purposes of Compact Research, a primary source consists of: 1) results of original research presented by an organization or researcher; 2) eyewitness accounts of events, personal experience, or work experience; 3) first-person editorials offering pundits' opinions; 4) government officials presenting political plans and/or policies; 5) representatives of organizations presenting testimony or policy.

❝There is a huge range of sports injuries. Some are serious enough to require medical attention and specialist treatment; others are relatively minor and respond to simple home care.❞

—Malcolm Read with Paul Wade, *Sports Injuries: A Unique Guide to Self-Diagnosis and Rehabilitation*. Philadelphia: Elsevier, 2009.

Read is a former Olympic athlete and now a medical advisor to the British Olympic association, and Wade is a sports journalist.

❝Traumatic injuries are, of course, very unpredictable. Sometimes they're due to poor conditioning, poor surfaces, or poor equipment. Oftentimes, they are just bad luck.❞

—Edward McFarland, interviewed by Charlene Laino, "Strains, Sprains, and Other Sports Injuries: Questions," WebMD, March 2010. webmd.com.

McFarland is team physician for the Johns Hopkins University Department of Athletics and for the Baltimore Orioles baseball team.

❝Football collisions may now be more dangerous to the brain than ever with the combination of bigger, stronger, and faster players and hard-shelled helmets that are often used as a weapon to initiate contact, creating a type of repetitive trauma to the brain that has never existed before.❞

—Christopher Nowinski, "Legal Issues Relating to Football Head Injuries," testimony to the US House Judiciary Committee, October 28, 2009. http://judiciary.house.gov.

Nowinski is codirector of the Center for the Study of Traumatic Encephalopathy at Boston University School of Medicine.

❝Winter sports injuries get a lot of attention at hospital emergency rooms, doctors' offices and clinics. Injuries include sprains and strains, dislocations and fractures.❞

—American Academy of Orthopaedic Surgeons, "Winter Sports Injury Prevention," July 2009. http://orthoinfo.aaos.org.

The American Academy of Orthopaedic Surgeons engages in health policy and advocacy activities on behalf of patients and the orthopedic surgery profession.

❝ Playing catch, shooting hoops, bicycling on a scenic path or just kicking around a soccer ball have more in common than you may think. On the up side, these activities are good exercise and are enjoyed by thousands of Americans. On the down side, they can result in a variety of injuries to the face. ❞

—American Academy of Otolaryngology—Head and Neck Surgery (AAO-HNS), "Facial Sports Injuries," July 21, 2011. www.entnet.org.

The AAO-HNS is composed of more than 12,000 specialists who treat the ear, nose, throat, and related structures of the head and neck.

❝ Sports concussions can be caused by colliding with another player, hitting the ground or other hard surface, or being hit by a piece of sports equipment. Concussions can even occur from body blows. Football players, for instance, can sustain concussions just from hits to the torso. ❞

—Cynthia Boyer, "Stay aHEAD of the Game: Get the Facts About Concussion in Sports," *Exceptional Parent*, March 2011.

Boyer is senior clinical director of Brain Injury Services at Bancroft, a nonprofit organization in Haddonfield, New Jersey, for people with neurological problems.

❝ Ice hockey catastrophic injuries usually occur when an athlete is struck from behind by an opponent, slides across the ice in a prone position, and makes contact with the crown of his/her head and the boards surrounding the rink. ❞

—Frederick O. Mueller and Robert C. Cantu, *Catastrophic Sports Injury Research: Twenty-Eighth Annual Report, Fall 1982– Spring 2010*, 2010. www.unc.edu.

Mueller is chair of the American Football Coaches Committee on Football Injuries, and Cantu is a Boston neurosurgeon and noted expert on sports-related concussions.

Facts and Illustrations

What Are Sports Injuries?

- The US Consumer Product Safety Commission consistently ranks **basketball, bicycling, baseball, soccer, and softball** (in that order) as the summer sports with the highest number of injuries.

- The American Association of Neurological Surgeons says that severe head trauma accounts for about **15 percent** of all injuries among skiers and snowboarders and is the most frequent cause of death and severe disability.

- According to the Mayo Clinic, people who have had a **concussion** double their risk of developing epilepsy within the first five years after the injury.

- Although body checking is not allowed in women's ice hockey, an examination of National Collegiate Athletic Association (NCAA) injury data revealed that concussions comprise **25 percent** of injuries in women's ice hockey, compared with **9 percent** in men's ice hockey.

- According to St. Louis, Missouri, orthopedic surgeon Rick Lehman, shoulder injuries account for about **20 percent** of all sports-related injuries.

- A 2010 report based on National Electronic Injury Surveillance System data showed that nearly half of all ankle injuries occurred during sports activities, with basketball the highest at **41 percent**, followed by football (9.3 percent), and soccer (8 percent).

Most Common Sports Injuries

Millions of people are treated in US emergency rooms each year for sports-related injuries ranging from minor cuts and bruises to broken bones and concussions. Common sports injuries include strains, sprains, and inflammation.

Sports Injury	Description	Caused By
Groin strain	Torn muscles in the upper thighs (adductors). Symptoms include sharp pain, swelling, and sometimes bruising.	A quick change in direction in sports such as football, soccer, volleyball, basketball, and tennis.
Runner's knee	Aches and pains in the knee from torn ligaments and cartilage. Accounts for over half of all sports injuries.	Running or jumping frequently, such as in running, cycling, football, soccer, basketball, and volleyball.
Shin splints	Inflammation and pain on the inner side of the shinbone.	Wearing worn-out shoes while running, workout increased too fast, and/or running and jumping on hard ground.
Shoulder injury (dislocation, sprains, strains)	Loosens the rotator cuff (the group of muscles and tendons that surround the shoulder) leading to pain, stiffness, weakness, and shoulder slippage. Accounts for 20 percent of all sports injuries.	Occurs during sports that involve lots of overhead use of the hands and arms, such as basketball.
Tendonitis	Inflammation of a tendon in various parts of the body (depending on the sport), including shoulders, elbows, wrists, hips, or the Achilles tendon, which connects the calf muscle to the heel bone.	Repeated stress and overuse, especially among athletes who golf, play tennis or baseball, swim, or participate in sports that involve running and jumping.
Ankle sprain	A tear in a tendon or ligament. Symptoms include pain, swelling, redness, and warmth at the injury site.	Running and turning quickly so the ankle twists, especially in sports such as hockey, soccer, basketball, football, and volleyball.

Source: Rick Lehman, "A Simple Guide to the Most Common Sports Injuries," May 17, 2011. http://drrick.org.

33

Most Head Injuries Occur in Cycling and Football

According to a July 2010 report by the American Association of Neurological Surgeons, nearly 450,000 sports-related head injuries were treated in US emergency rooms during 2009, with the highest number in cycling and football.

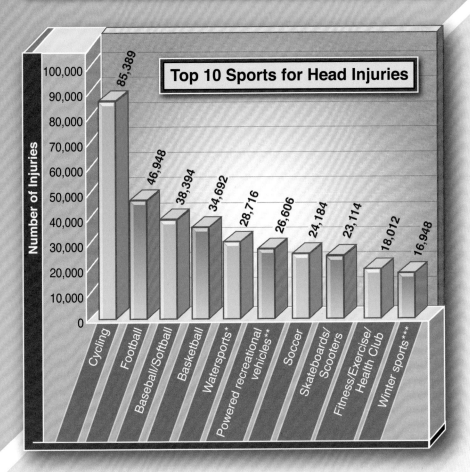

Top 10 Sports for Head Injuries

Number of Injuries

- Cycling: 85,389
- Football: 46,948
- Baseball/Softball: 38,394
- Basketball: 34,692
- Watersports*: 28,716
- Powered recreational vehicles**: 26,606
- Soccer: 24,184
- Skateboards/Scooters: 23,114
- Fitness/Exercise/Health Club: 18,012
- Winter sports***: 16,948

* Water sports include diving, scuba diving, surfing, swimming, water polo, water skiing, and water tubing.

** Power recreational vehicles include ATVs, dune buggies, go-carts, mini bikes, and off-road vehicles.

*** Winter sports include skiing, sledding, snowboarding, and snowmobiling.

Source: American Association of Neurological Surgeons, "Sports-Related Head Injury," July 2010. http://mobile.aans.org.

Most Concussions Affect Teen Athletes

According to a 2011 report based on data from the Healthcare Cost and Utilization Project, approximately 44,000 visits to US emergency departments in 2008 were related to concussions sustained during sports activities. Over half of these concussions affected teenagers.

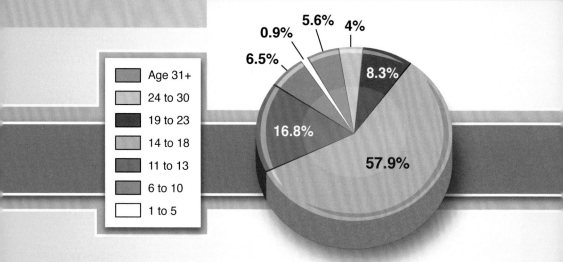

Legend:
- Age 31+
- 24 to 30
- 19 to 23
- 14 to 18
- 11 to 13
- 6 to 10
- 1 to 5

0.9%
5.6%
4%
6.5%
8.3%
16.8%
57.9%

Source: Lan Zhao, Weiwei Han, and Claudia Steiner, "Sports Related Concussions, 2008," H-CUP *Statistical Brief #114*, May 2011. www.hcup-us.ahrq.gov.

- According to the Sports Concussion Institute, as many as **3.8 million** sports- and recreation-related concussions occur in the United States each year.

- The American Academy of Orthopaedic Surgeons states that each year, over **63,000** hockey-related injuries are serious enough to require medical attention.

- According to the American Association of Neurological Surgeons, sports that saw substantial increases in injuries from 2008 to 2009 include **water sports, cycling, baseball and softball, and basketball** (in that order).

How Serious a Problem Are Injuries in Youth Sports?

❝Contact sports have inherent dangers that put young athletes at special risk for severe injuries. Even with rigorous training and proper safety equipment, youngsters are still at risk for severe injuries to the neck, spinal cord, and growth plates.❞

—NIAMS, an agency of the National Institutes of Health that supports research into diseases of (and injuries to) bones, joints, muscles, and skin.

❝I'm skeptical that athletes really understand the dangers. In this week alone I have had two high-level athletes in different sports ask me if they can play after recent concussions despite the fact that they are both still having symptoms.❞

—David Geier, an orthopedic surgeon and director of the Sports Medicine Program at the Medical University of South Carolina.

By the time Lucy Gonzalez was 16 years old, she had suffered six concussions—and the last one ended her soccer career. A standout athlete for Jerome High School in Dublin, Ohio, Gonzalez had a passion for soccer, and she pushed herself hard whenever she played. If her head was aching she told no one, as she did not want to take the chance of having the coaches sideline her. Gonzalez's sixth concussion oc-

curred during a spring 2010 championship game when she was slammed in the head by a soccer ball. As she stumbled off the field, her mind was foggy, her vision was blurred, and she was unable to understand what her coaches and teammates were saying to her. As young as she was, her reign as a soccer star was over. "When I lost soccer," she says, "I lost my friends. I lost what I loved. I lost the life I worked so hard to get."[25]

Rather than giving in to despair, Gonzalez opted to use her experience to help other young athletes. She attends soccer matches, and when players insist on getting back in the game after they have been hurt, the coach sends them to talk to her. Gonzalez is frank about what she went through, making it clear that the same thing could happen to them. She describes the effects of brain damage that still plague her, including bouts of depression, uncontrollable crying jags, dizzy spells, and memory loss. She also emphasizes that having to give up her beloved sport is no one's fault but her own. "Soccer did not put me in this situation," she says. "Thinking I could play no matter how much I hurt is what did."[26] And when Gonzalez tells kids that, they listen.

A Spike in Youth Concussions

Gonzalez's story is not uncommon, as research shows that concussion rates are high among young athletes and are increasing. This trend is a serious concern for health officials and was the focus of a study that was published in the August 30, 2010, issue of *Pediatrics*. Conducted by researchers from Providence, Rhode Island, the study found that from 1997 to 2007, concussions among athletes aged 8 to 13 doubled—and among older teens they tripled. Says Lisa Bakhos, a pediatric emergency physician at Jersey Shore University Medical Center and the study's lead researcher: "Many parents, coaches, teachers, and other adults feel that, because these athletes are so young, they could not possibly get seriously hurt. As we have seen time and time again, this is of course not the case."[27]

One sport that has been associated with an alarming number of concussions among girls is basketball. A 2010 study by the National

> **One sport that has been associated with an alarming number of concussions among girls is basketball.**

> **Injuries are an unfortunate fact of life for athletes of all ages, no matter what sport they play. What has health officials concerned, though, is that youth sports injuries are rising at an alarming rate.**

Athletic Trainers' Association examined concussions among high school basketball players and found that incidence among females was 240 percent higher than males. Mikayla Wilson, a 14-year-old girl from Spangle, Washington, sustained a concussion during a basketball game in February 2011. After being knocked to the gym floor by a player on the opposing team, Wilson got up and noticed that her head hurt. Since she did not appear to be injured, her coaches kept her in the game—but when it was over, people could see that something was seriously wrong. Wilson turned to her mother, pointed to her teammates, and asked: "Who are those girls dressed just like I am and why are they looking at me?"[28]

Wilson was taken to a hospital where she underwent a CT scan. The test ruled out a skull fracture and bleeding inside the brain, so doctors concluded that she had a concussion. A few weeks after being injured Wilson's memory was starting to return, and doctors were fairly confident that she would make a full recovery.

Kids Pushed Too Hard

Injuries are an unfortunate fact of life for athletes of all ages, no matter what sport they play. What has health officials concerned, though, is that youth sports injuries are rising at an alarming rate. Thomas M. DeBerardino, an orthopedic surgeon who specializes in sports medicine, refers to this trend as a "silent epidemic." According to DeBerardino, when kids are overscheduled and not urged to take time off between sports, injuries are much more likely to happen. "More adolescents are participating in year-round sports without seasonal breaks," he says, "or they are playing on multiple teams simultaneously. This increased exposure means there will continue to be growing numbers of significant musculoskeletal injuries, both traumatic and chronic overuse."[29]

Overuse injuries in young athletes appear to be more prevalent in

some sports than others. Baseball, for instance, has a high rate of overuse injuries, especially among pitchers. This was revealed in a study published in March 2011 by the American Sports Medicine Institute, which involved 481 baseball players aged 9 to 14. The group found that kids who pitched more than 100 innings in a year were 3.5 times more likely to be injured than those who pitched fewer innings. Says lead researcher Glenn S. Fleisig:

> It is a tough balancing act for adults to give their young athletes as much opportunity as possible to develop skills and strength without exposing them to increased risk of overuse injury. Based on this study, we recommend that pitchers in high school and younger pitch no more than 100 innings in competition in any calendar year. Some pitchers need to be limited even more, because no pitcher should continue to pitch when fatigued.[30]

Kent Myer is very familiar with the anguish caused by an overuse injury. A star pitcher on his high school baseball team in Jackson, Alabama, Myer first began to notice pain in his right arm in April 2007 when he was a junior. He did not think too much about it, and even when the pain kept getting worse he continued to play. "Being the competitor that I am," he says, "I played through the pain. I would simply take 800 milligrams of Ibuprofen before I was scheduled to pitch and be fine."[31] Myer was not fine, however, as he learned during his senior year. The state championships had just begun, and he was on the pitcher's mound when he suddenly found that he could not throw the ball. "I felt something in my elbow give and my pitch went a mere 20 feet," he says. "The feeling was a weird one. It was as if all my strength in my elbow was suddenly taken away. I tried to throw another pitch thinking nothing was wrong, but I had the same result."[32]

Two weeks later, Myer had an MRI and doctors found that he had suffered a tear in his right ulnar collateral ligament (UCL), which is the main stabilizing ligament in the elbow. The following June he had UCL reconstructive surgery, and then underwent intense physical therapy for the next eight months. But the hardest part was being sidelined during his freshman year at Alabama State University, rather than pitching for the school's Crimson Tide baseball team, which had long been Myer's

dream. "It was difficult being injured," he says. "To sit out and watch everyone else play was a hard thing to go through."[33]

Cheerleading

There was a time when cheerleaders were known for cheering, rather than performing acrobatics. They stood in front of the crowd, doing jumps and kicks, yelling through megaphones to inspire their team, and had little or no risk of injury. That, however, is no longer the case. With highly publicized national competitions and the pressure to perform fancier, trickier, and riskier stunts, cheerleading has become the most dangerous sport for female athletes. This was revealed in a 2009 study by the National Center for Catastrophic Sports Injury Research, which found that cheerleading accounts for 65 percent of all catastrophic injuries in girls' high school athletics. Says the group's director, Frederick Mueller: "Cheerleading has changed dramatically, from females jumping up and down and shaking pom-poms to a gymnastics-type event where they're throwing girls 25–30 feet in the air—and sometimes missing them on the way down."[34]

> With highly publicized national competitions and the pressure to perform fancier, trickier, and riskier stunts, cheerleading has become the most dangerous sport for female athletes.

Alexa McCormack suffered three concussions during her time as a cheerleader at West Milford High School in Passaic County, New Jersey. The second one happened during her junior year when she was performing at a competition. A teammate fell from nearly 10 feet (3m) in the air and crashed into the side of McCormack's head, knocking her unconscious and splitting her eardrum. McCormack was treated at a hospital but began to suffer from blurred vision, memory loss, and migraine headaches. She was sidelined for eight months, and then returned to competition for her senior year—only to sustain a third concussion less than a month later. Now McCormack's cheerleading days are over, and she can no longer participate in any kind of contact sport. "Knowing I'm not allowed to do anything ever again

stinks," she says. "When you break your leg, it heals and you can tumble again. But with the brain, there's nothing you can ever do about it."[35]

Sudden Death

Accounts of young people who die suddenly while playing or practicing sports are tragic and heartbreaking, but these deaths are rare. Health officials say that when a young athlete collapses and dies after physical exertion, the most likely cause is an undiagnosed heart condition that leads to sudden cardiac arrest. According to cardiologist Ronald Grifka, this occurs only in about 1 out of every 200,000 athletes, and he has only seen 3 or 4 cases in 20 years. "It's an uncommon finding," he says. "Millions of kids play sports and have no problem at all."[36]

As rare as sudden cardiac arrest may be, that is no consolation for the grief-stricken families of young athletes who have died from it. Gary and Jocelyn Leonard, who live in the southern Michigan town of Fennville, are very familiar with the devastation of losing someone to sudden cardiac arrest because it claimed their son's life. During a basketball game on March 3, 2011, in front of a cheering crowd, 16-year-old Wes Leonard made the winning basket in overtime and clinched his team's perfect 20–0 season—and then seconds later collapsed on the gym floor. He was rushed to the hospital where doctors tried to resuscitate him for over two hours, but they were unable to save him. An autopsy later showed that Wes had an enlarged heart that was never diagnosed, and he had died from cardiac arrest. "We didn't understand," says his mother. "How can that happen to the biggest, strongest, healthiest kid in your school? I think you can't comprehend that the heart can stop."[37]

> **As rare as sudden cardiac arrest may be, that is no consolation for the grief-stricken families of young athletes who have died from it.**

Heatstroke is even rarer than sudden cardiac arrest, but its prevalence appears to be growing. According to Andrew Grundstein, an associate professor at the University of Georgia, sudden death from heatstroke among youth has increased from about 1 death per year in the 1980s to an average of 2.8

deaths per year. Grundstein theorizes that this spike is due to record heat waves, combined with the fact that high school players are bigger than in the past—and often overweight.

One heatstroke victim was 16-year-old Tyler Davenport, who attended high school in Lamar, Arkansas. After football practice on a blazing-hot August day in 2010, Davenport collapsed on the ground. His coaches wrapped him in ice towels in an effort to cool him down, but by the time paramedics got him to the hospital, his temperature had climbed to a deadly 108.5°F (42.5°C). Over the next two months, Davenport's condition continued to deteriorate until his liver, pancreas, and kidneys were no longer functioning. On October 12, 2010, the young athlete died.

Youth at Risk

Sports injuries are a serious problem among young people, and studies show that the problem is getting worse. Most of these injuries are relatively minor, such as sprains, strains, and tired muscles, but others can result in lifelong damage, the abrupt end of a sports career, and even death. With more and more youth becoming involved in sports each year, the number of injuries will likely keep growing. Through increased awareness of sports injuries, along with better diagnostic and prevention methods, this trend can hopefully be slowed in the future.

How Serious a Problem Are Injuries in Youth Sports?

"Sports injuries are the most common type of injury in adolescents, and sports-related injury is the leading reason for adolescent visits to primary care providers."

—Mark D. Miller, Jennifer Adele Hart, John M. MacKnight, *Essential Orthopaedics*. Philadelphia: Saunders Elsevier, 2009.

Miller and MacKnight are orthopedic surgeons, and Hart is a physician assistant.

....

"While much focus has been given to players in the National Football League (NFL), it is important to remember that high school athletes represent the single largest segment of football players in the country and account for the majority of sport-related concussions."

—Michael Prybicien, "Protecting School-Age Athletes from Sports-Related Concussion Injury," congressional hearing, House Energy and Commerce Committee, September 8, 2010. http://democrats.energycommerce.house.gov.

Prybicien is head athletic trainer at Passaic High School in Clifton, New Jersey, and president of the Athletic Trainer Society of New Jersey.

....

* Editor's Note: While the definition of a primary source can be narrowly or broadly defined, for the purposes of Compact Research, a primary source consists of: 1) results of original research presented by an organization or researcher; 2) eyewitness accounts of events, personal experience, or work experience; 3) first-person editorials offering pundits' opinions; 4) government officials presenting political plans and/or policies; 5) representatives of organizations presenting testimony or policy.

✨ **Regardless of whether most injuries are intentional or not, the sad and harsh reality is that minor hockey is plagued with a serious injury factor and bodychecking is responsible for a disproportionately large number of those injuries, including concussions.** ✨

—Emile J. Therien, "Injuries in Minor Hockey—Study by Researchers from the University of Buffalo," *British Journal of Sports Medicine*, August 12, 2010. http://bjsm.bmj.com.

Therien is a public health and safety advocate and past president of the Canada Safety Council in Ottawa, Ontario, Canada.

✨ **Playing sports is wonderful for children and adolescents, but moderation is very important. If stress fractures are detected too late in child and adolescent athletes, they pose a risk of true fracture, deformity or growth disturbance requiring surgical treatment.** ✨

—Alison Field, "Prevent Stress Fractures in Kids—Cross Train and Don't Specialize Early," *STOP Sports Injuries* (blog), June 22, 2011. www.stopsportsinjuries.org.

Field is associate professor of pediatrics at Children's Hospital Boston.

✨ **Head trauma is one of the most common injuries sustained by young athletes. . . . The consequences can include impaired intellectual abilities, severe neurological disorders and other long-term disabilities.** ✨

—Cynthia Boyer, "Stay aHEAD of the Game: Get the Facts About Concussion in Sports," *Exceptional Parent*, March 2011.

Boyer is senior clinical director of Brain Injury Services at Bancroft, a nonprofit organization in Haddonfield, New Jersey, for people with neurological problems.

✨ **Cheerleader falls from gymnastic-type stunts have been reported to have a greater impact than being tackled by a professional football player.** ✨

—US Sports Academy, "Cheerleading Ranks First in Catastrophic Sports Injuries," April 2011. www.ussa.edu.

The US Sports Academy is a sports university located in Daphne, Alabama.

"The bones, muscles, tendons, ligaments and joints are not fully developed until the end of puberty. . . . Because sports injury or pain in these 'growth sites' can lead to permanent injury, persistent pain around joints should never be ignored or dismissed as 'growing pains.'"

—Palo Alto Medical Foundation, "Sports Injuries," 2011. www.pamf.org.

The Palo Alto Medical Foundation specializes in medical care, biomedical research, and education.

"Sometimes people believe that it shows strength and courage to play when you're injured. Not only is that belief wrong, it can put a young athlete at risk for serious injury."

—CDC, "Cole's Story," *Injury Center Connection Newsletter*, Spring/Summer 2011. www.cdc.gov.

As the premier public health agency in the United States, the CDC conducts and supports a wide array of health-related activities and research.

"Children and adolescent athletes are also at particularly high risk of experiencing second-impact syndrome, a condition that occurs when an athlete who has sustained an initial head injury sustains a second head injury before the symptoms associated with the first have fully cleared."

—Joel S. Brenner, "Protecting School-Age Athletes from Sports-Related Concussion Injury," congressional hearing, House Energy and Commerce Committee, September 8, 2010. http://democrats.energycommerce.house.gov.

Brenner is medical director of the Sports Medicine Program at Children's Hospital of the King's Daughters in Norfolk, Virginia, and associate professor of pediatrics at Eastern Virginia Medical School.

How Serious a Problem Are Injuries in Youth Sports?

- According to the American College of Emergency Physicians, over **3.5 million** kids 14 and under are treated for sports-related injuries each year.

- The CDC says that high school athletes suffer **2 million** injuries each year, of which 500,000 are serious enough to warrant doctor visits and 20,000 require hospitalization.

- Data from the Center for Injury Research and Policy at Nationwide Children's Hospital show that as many as **40 percent** of high school athletes who sustain concussions return to sports prematurely, which raises the risk for more severe head injuries.

- According to the National Athletic Trainers' Association, there are five times as many **catastrophic football injuries** among high school athletes as college athletes.

- According to Safe Kids USA, **715,000** sports- and recreation-related injuries occur each year in school settings alone.

- According to the American Academy of Ophthalmology, sports involvement is the most common cause of **eye injury** among children aged 5 to 14.

Most Common Injuries in High School Athletes

According to researchers from the Center for Injury Research and Policy, involvement in high school sports has soared from about 4 million participants in 1971 to over 7 million in 2011. While participation in athletics is highly beneficial for young people, injuries are inevitable. The most common injuries sustained by high school athletes while practicing or competing during the 2010–2011 school year were strains and sprains.

Injuries during practice

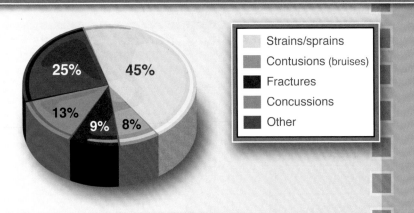

Strains/sprains
Contusions (bruises)
Fractures
Concussions
Other

Injuries during competition

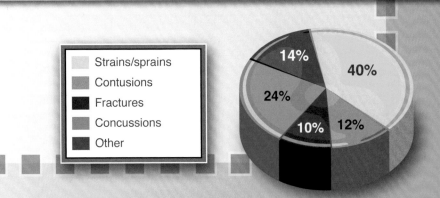

Strains/sprains
Contusions
Fractures
Concussions
Other

Note: Represents injuries that occurred as a result of participation in an organized high school competition, practice, or performance that required medical attention by a team physician, certified athletic trainer, personal physician, or emergency department/urgent care facility.

Source: R. Dawn Comstock, Christy L. Collins, and Natalie McIlvain, *National High School Sports-Related Injury Surveillance Study: 2010–2011 School Year,* 2011. http://injuryresearch.net.

Cheerleading Most Dangerous Sport for Girls

According to a report by Frederick O. Mueller and Robert C. Cantu of the National Center for Catastrophic Sports Injury Research, of 11 sports that are most popular with high school girls, cheerleading causes the highest number of serious and catastrophic injuries, including permanent paralysis and death.

Serious and Catastrophic Injuries Among Female High School Athletes, 1982 to 2010

Sport	Fatality	Nonfatal	Serious
Cheerleading	2	28	48
Gymnastics	0	6	3
Track	1	2	6
Swimming	0	4	1
Basketball	0	1	3
Ice Hockey	0	0	2
Field Hockey	0	3	0
Softball	1	2	2
Lacrosse	0	0	2
Soccer	0	1	2
Volleyball	0	1	0

Source: Frederick O. Mueller and Robert C. Cantu, *Catastrophic Sports Injury Report: Twenty-Eighth Annual Report, Fall 1982–Spring 2010*, June 2011. www.unc.edu.

- The American Association of Neurological Surgeons says that sports and recreational activities contribute to **21 percent** of all traumatic brain injuries among American children and adolescents.

Rare Sudden Death in Teen Athletes

Sudden death during youth sports activities is a rare occurrence. To examine the causes of sudden death, researchers analyzed 1,866 deaths that occurred between 1980 and 2006 involving young athletes in competitive sports. The researchers found that over 50 percent of the deaths were caused by heart problems.

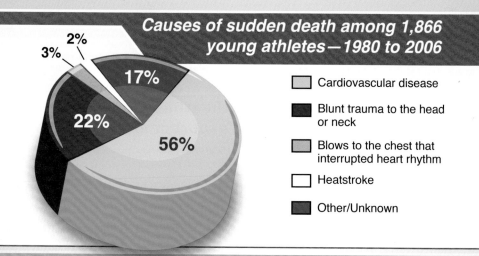

Causes of sudden death among 1,866 young athletes—1980 to 2006

- 2%
- 3%
- 17%
- 22%
- 56%

- ☐ Cardiovascular disease
- ■ Blunt trauma to the head or neck
- ▨ Blows to the chest that interrupted heart rhythm
- ☐ Heatstroke
- ■ Other/Unknown

Source: Barry J. Maron et al. "Sudden Deaths in Young Competitive Athletes: Analysis of 1866 Deaths in the United States, 1980–2006," *Circulation: Journal of the American Heart Association*, February 16, 2009.

- A study released in 2010 by researchers from Ohio found that basketball-related traumatic brain injuries among adolescents increased **70 percent** between 1997 and 2007.

- According to the STOP Sports Injuries campaign, the number of serious **shoulder and elbow injuries** among youth baseball and softball players has increased fivefold since 2000.

- The CDC says that for young people aged 15 to 24, sports are second only to motor vehicle accidents as the leading cause of **brain injury**.

How Are Sports Injuries Treated?

"There is often more than one way to effectively treat an injury. Treatment programs are always adjusted to meet the individual needs of the athlete and the unique requirements of the athlete's sport or activity."

—American Academy of Pediatrics, which is composed of 60,000 physicians who specialize in pediatric medicine.

"Today, the outlook for an injured athlete is far more optimistic than in the past. Sports medicine has developed some near-miraculous ways to help athletes heal and, in most cases, return to sports."

—NIAMS, an agency of the National Institutes of Health that supports research into diseases of (and injuries to) bones, joints, muscles, and skin.

On June 12, 2011, 19-year-old Connor Docherty finished walking Scotland's famed West Highland Way, a long-distance footpath that winds through 96 miles (154.5km) of scenic countryside. Since tens of thousands of people make the journey every year, Docherty's trek may seem unremarkable. But it was an amazing achievement because three years before, he had been badly injured during a rugby game and left paralyzed from the neck down.

When the accident happened, Docherty was in his second year at St. Aloysius' College in Glasgow, Scotland. During a January 2008 match against Edinburgh Academy, something went terribly wrong when he tackled an opponent. "It was a freak accident," he says. "I made a tackle on my opposite number and my head was in the wrong position at the time.

I blacked out and, when I came round, I was lying on the pitch [field] but I wasn't in any pain. It was really quite surreal because I couldn't feel anything from the shoulders down."[38] Docherty was taken to the hospital, and tests showed that he had broken three vertebrae in his neck and damaged his spinal cord. In an operation that lasted more than 11 hours, doctors fused his vertebrae back together using a bone graft from his hip and a metal known as titanium. But there was nothing they could do to fix his spinal cord, and they warned Docherty that he might never walk again.

Unwilling to Give Up

Docherty was determined to prove the doctors wrong. After his surgery, he began the long, grueling process of rehabilitation with the help of a hospital physical therapist. Gradually he began to notice that feeling was returning to his arms and then to his legs, which fueled his motivation to overcome his disability. "It was hard going, doing rehab every day," he says. "It could be exhausting but I just wanted to keep going. There were moments of frustration but they were fleeting and you just have to deal with it."[39]

And deal with it he did. Six months after he was injured, Docherty walked out of the hospital on crutches. Although he knew that he would not be able to play rugby again, the progress he had made motivated him to work even harder. To build up his strength, he worked out on gym equipment at home, and in September 2010 he teamed up with physical therapist Eilidh Dorrian. They got together three or four times a week for sessions that lasted two hours, including a 30-minute walk, and once a month they walked 5 miles (8k). In the beginning Docherty had painful cramps and spasms in his legs,

> "A crucial part of rehabilitation is exercise that starts slowly and becomes more challenging over time, which is known as a graduated exercise program."

but over time those went away and walking became easier for him. Seeing his incredible progress inspired Dorrian to suggest that they set a long-term goal: to walk the West Highland Way.

Their trek was not without challenges, as it was a very long distance for Docherty to walk and the weather was windy and rainy during the entire six days. But at the end, he was thrilled to have finished and proud of himself, as were Dorrian and numerous others. Dominic McKay, who is an executive with the organization Scottish Rugby, offered hearty congratulations to Docherty, calling what he had done a "tremendous achievement." Says McKay: "Connor is a truly inspirational young man."[40]

Surgery Versus Rehabilitation

Docherty's accomplishment is a powerful testimony to how fierce determination and hard work can help an athlete recover after a serious sports injury. As he learned, a crucial part of rehabilitation is exercise that starts slowly and becomes more challenging over time, which is known as a graduated exercise program. According to the NIAMS, a complete rehabilitation program should include exercises that build flexibility, endurance, and strength, as the group explains: "As damaged tissue heals, scar tissue forms, which shrinks and brings torn or separated tissues back together. As a result, the injury site becomes tight or stiff, and damaged tissues are at risk of reinjury. That's why stretching and strengthening exercises are so important."[41]

A study published in July 2010 by researchers from Sweden and Denmark found that rehabilitation works as well as surgery in young, active adults who have sustained ACL injuries. The 121 participants ranged in age from 18 to 35 and were all nonprofessional athletes who had torn an ACL while playing sports. Roughly half of the group had ACL repair surgery immediately, and the rest participated in a physical therapy program for two years. At the

> " Orthopedic surgeons widely believe that one of the most promising treatments for sports injuries is arthroscopic surgery (also known as arthroscopy), a technique that allows a surgeon to view joint problems and correct them without performing an invasive operation. "

end of the study, both groups reported substantial improvement, and the researchers found no significant differences in pain or ability to function between the groups. The study authors write:

> Our findings indicate that in young, active adults with an acute ACL tear, a strategy of structured rehabilitation plus early ACL reconstruction did not result in better patient-reported outcomes at 2 years than a strategy of rehabilitation. . . . With the use of the latter strategy, more than half the ACL reconstructions could be avoided without adversely affecting outcomes.[42]

Although studies such as this one show that rehabilitation is a viable option for athletes, most choose to undergo ACL surgery because it allows them to return to their sport sooner. That is a concern for some physicians, who say that it vastly increases the athletes' chances of developing serious problems later in life. One of the biggest risks is osteoarthritis, which occurs when cartilage in the knee wears away and the bone becomes exposed, causing the unprotected joint surfaces to rub against each other.

When an athlete sustains an ACL injury, both the ligament itself and cartilage are damaged—but unlike the ACL, cartilage does not heal or regenerate. Thus, as stress continues to be placed on the injured knee during sports, the risk of osteoarthritis increases. Dr. Robert Stanton, who is president of the American Orthopaedic Society for Sports Medicine, says that even when young athletes are told about this risk, almost all still choose to have the ACL surgically repaired. He explains: "They're young, they're invulnerable. Above all, they just want to keep playing."[43]

Minimal Invasiveness, Maximum Benefits

Orthopedic surgeons widely believe that one of the most promising treatments for sports injuries is arthroscopic surgery (also known as arthroscopy), a technique that allows a surgeon to view joint problems and correct them without performing an invasive operation. During an arthroscopy, the surgeon makes a tiny cut in the skin and then uses an instrument known as an arthroscope to examine the insides of joints. The American Orthopaedic Society for Sports Medicine explains: "The tiny lens and fiber optic light of the arthroscope is connected to a camera

and monitor that allows the orthopaedic surgeon to see inside the joint and perform a variety of different procedures."[44]

Guided by the magnified image of the joint, a surgeon can repair damaged tissue with surgical instruments inserted through small incisions in the skin. The NIAMS writes: "Using arthroscopy, for example, a surgeon may reattach the torn ends of a ligament or reconstruct the ligament by using a piece (graft) of healthy ligament from the patient or from a cadaver."[45] The group adds that because arthroscopy uses tiny incisions, it results in less pain, swelling, and scarring than conventional surgery and thus decreases rehabilitation time. Another advantage is that most arthroscopies can be performed on an outpatient basis, so patients do not have to spend time in the hospital.

> " A study released in July 2010 found that athletes who undergo arthroscopic surgery for hip injuries have an excellent chance of being able to return to sports at their preinjury level of ability. "

A study released in July 2010 found that athletes who undergo arthroscopic surgery for hip injuries have an excellent chance of being able to return to sports at their preinjury level of ability. Researchers from Rush University Medical Center in Chicago focused on those who suffered from a condition known as femoral acetabular impingement (FAI), which involves damage to the ball and socket joint of the hip. Lead investigator Shane J. Nho explains: "Many athletes experience early on-set of symptoms of FAI because . . . their athletic activities require a high degree of motion and force through the joint. Symptoms of FAI . . . include pain, limited range of motion, and for athletes, loss of the ability to compete at their top level."[46]

Nho and his team identified 47 athletes, all of whom were diagnosed with FAI. These were a mix of high school, college, and professional athletes from a wide variety of sports, including ice and field hockey, soccer, baseball, swimming, lacrosse, football, tennis, running, and horseback riding. All participants underwent arthroscopic surgery for their FAI injuries and were then tracked for 16 months so their progress could be as-

sessed. The team found that 78 percent of the athletes were able to return to their sport within an average of 9 months following the procedure, and over 90 percent were able to compete at the same level as they had before being injured.

Recognizing Concussions

Unlike most sports injuries, no treatment exists specifically for concussions. The only remedy is mental and physical rest, as orthopedic surgeon and sports medicine specialist Michael Stuart writes: "Treatment should include a period of both physical rest and cognitive rest following the concussion to give the brain time to heal. Return to sports should be gradual after all symptoms have cleared. An athlete who has had a concussion shouldn't return to a contact sport like hockey until a health care provider has given approval."[47] Yet one of the biggest problems associated with concussions begins long before a doctor orders a patient to rest. The initial challenge is being able to tell whether an athlete has sustained a concussion. This is especially true at schools that have no certified athletic trainer on staff—and according to a Scripps Howard News Service report, that applies to most schools.

In August 2010 the group released a four-month review showing that barely a third of America's high schools with a sports program employed a full-time athletic trainer. The absence of such a qualified professional puts a great deal of pressure on coaches and others who are not trained in recognizing the signs of concussions. Many do not know, for instance, that the majority of concussion sufferers never lose consciousness and may look and act as though nothing is wrong. Says Julian Bailes, who is director of the Brain Injury Research Institute, an NCAA team physician, and a former physician for the NFL: "With the vast majority of concussions in sports—90 percent of the time, in fact—athletes don't get knocked out. They're walking around and talking, and they look normal."[48]

> " Unlike most sports injuries, no treatment exists specifically for concussions. The only remedy is mental and physical rest. "

Because of the challenges involved in being able to tell if an athlete has suffered a concussion, it is critical for athletic personnel to have tools that can measure athletes' brain functions immediately after injuries. To address this need, Cleveland Clinic biomedical engineer Jay Alberts developed an application for the Apple iPad 2 that features two sections: one that tests cognitive abilities and another that tests physical abilities. In the first part of the screening, athletes answer questions that test their reaction time, memory, and thinking skills. During the second part, the iPad is strapped onto an athlete's waist to measure balance and stability on soft and hard surfaces.

As of August 2011 Alberts and his team were involved in a pilot study to test the new technology at two Northeastern Ohio high schools and one university. The 100 participants in the study included male football players, female and male soccer players, and female volleyball players, who were all deemed high risk based on their sport and the positions they played. Says Don McPhillips, who is head athletic trainer at the college involved in the study: "I think of it as another tool in the tool belt. Trying to identify concussions is tough."[49]

Rehab, Repair, Rebound

Although sports injuries are extremely common, a number of treatments can help athletes recover from them. Rehabilitation builds muscle, strength, and endurance, while arthroscopy can repair damaged tissue and save an athlete from having to undergo major surgery. With new computer tools being developed, those who have sustained concussions may be diagnosed early enough that severe brain damage can be avoided. As research continues, scientists will undoubtedly create even better treatment methods that help athletes recover quickly and get back to their positions on the field, the court, the rink, or anywhere else they play their favorite sports.

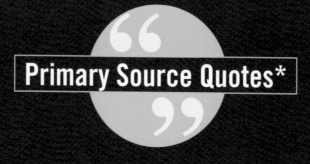

Primary Source Quotes*

How Are Sports Injuries Treated?

❝ Priorities, commitment, fitness, and conditioning levels contribute to how fast an athlete is ready to return to the playing field. ❞

—Christine M. MacDonell, "Teamwork Between Patients and Therapists Is Central to Sports Medicine," *Newsweek*, February 2, 2010. www.newsweekshowcase.com.

MacDonell is the managing director of medical rehabilitation with CARF International, an independent accreditor of health and human services.

❝ Most commonly applied to the knee, shoulder, ankle, elbow, and hip, arthroscopy is the gold-standard tool for definitive diagnosis and treatment of joint-related injuries. ❞

—Sam W. Wiesel and John N. Delahay, eds., *Essentials of Orthopedic Surgery*. New York: Springer, 2010.

Wiesel and Delahay are physicians with the Department of Orthopaedic Surgery at Georgetown University Medical Center.

* Editor's Note: While the definition of a primary source can be narrowly or broadly defined, for the purposes of Compact Research, a primary source consists of: 1) results of original research presented by an organization or researcher; 2) eyewitness accounts of events, personal experience, or work experience; 3) first-person editorials offering pundits' opinions; 4) government officials presenting political plans and/or policies; 5) representatives of organizations presenting testimony or policy.

> **Rest is the best way to allow your brain to recover from a concussion. . . . This means avoiding general physical exertion as well as activities that require mental concentration, such as playing video games, watching TV, texting or using a computer. School workloads should also be temporarily reduced.**

—Mayo Clinic, "Concussion: Treatments and Drugs," February 22, 2011. www.mayoclinic.com.

The Mayo Clinic is a world-renowned medical facility headquartered in Rochester, Minnesota.

> **The key to the treatment of stress fractures is early recognition. If recognized early, most stress fractures will heal fully with activity restriction.**

—Alison Field, "Prevent Stress Fractures in Kids—Cross Train and Don't Specialize Early," *STOP Sports Injuries*, (blog), June 22, 2011. www.stopsportsinjuries.org.

Field is an associate professor of pediatrics at Children's Hospital Boston.

> **Left untreated, throwing injuries in the elbow can become complicated conditions.**

—American Academy of Orthopaedic Surgeons, "Throwing Injuries in the Elbow in Children," April 2011. http://orthoinfo.aaos.org.

The American Academy of Orthopaedic Surgeons engages in health policy and advocacy activities on behalf of patients and the orthopedic surgery profession.

> **The most obvious treatment for overuse is rest, especially from the activity that created the injury in the first place. Ice is also used to reduce soreness and inflammation.**

—American Orthopaedic Society for Sports Medicine, "Overuse Injuries in Baseball/Softball," *AOSSM Sports Tips*, 2009. www.sportsmed.org.

Composed of over 3,000 physicians and other health professionals, the society serves as a forum for education and research.

❝Brain cells should be left to rest days to weeks following a concussion and should not be subjected to any type of intellectual stimulation.❞

—Bennet I. Omalu, *Head and Other Injuries in Youth, High School, College and Professional Football*, statement to the US House of Representatives, Brain Injury Research Institute, February 1, 2010. www.braininjuryresearchinstitute.org.

Omalu is a physician and codirector of the Brain Injury Research Institute at West Virginia University in Morgantown, West Virginia.

❝Sometimes that 'sprain' is actually an ankle fracture and treatment[s] for these two conditions are very different. And don't skimp on rehab! An ankle that has not been properly healed and strengthened is more likely to suffer repeated sprains, leading to chronic ankle instability.❞

—American College of Foot and Ankle Surgeons, "Foot Health Facts for Athletes," September 30, 2010. www.foothealthfacts.org.

The American College of Foot and Ankle Surgeons represents over 6,000 podiatrists with specialty training in surgical and nonsurgical treatment of conditions of the foot and ankle.

Facts and Illustrations

How Are Sports Injuries Treated?

- According to Safe Kids USA, over **3.5 million** children aged 14 and under receive medical treatment for sports injuries each year.

- The American Association of Neurological Surgeons says that **10 to 15 percent** of high school athletes sustain concussions each year, and only a fraction receives proper treatment.

- According to the CDC, **16 percent** of all unintentional injuries treated in hospital emergency departments each year are the result of injuries from sports and recreational activities.

- St. Louis, Missouri, orthopedic surgeon Rick Lehman says that runner's knee, which can result from any sport that involves running and jumping, comprises **25 percent** of all orthopedic surgeries.

- According to the STOP Sports Injuries campaign, rehabilitation after a **wrestling injury** is an important part of preventing further injury, since a large number of all injuries result from aggravation of an old one.

- Exercise physiologist Elizabeth Quinn says that a **severed Achilles tendon** requires surgery and up to 12 weeks in a cast.

- According to the NIAMS, if severe strains are not treated professionally, **permanent damage** and **loss of function** can result.

Rehabilitation and Healing

According to the National Institute of Arthritis and Musculoskeletal and Skin Diseases, a variety of tactics can help athletes recover from sports injuries.

Therapy	Description	Desired Result
Rest	Although an injured athlete should get moving again as soon as possible, rest following an injury is also important.	Proper rest helps promote healing
Electrostimulation	Mild electrical current prevents nerve cells from sending pain impulses to the brain and can also cause muscles in immobilized limbs to contract.	Relieves pain, decreases swelling, helps prevent muscle atrophy and weakness
Cold/Cryotherapy	Ice packs cause blood vessels to constrict and limit blood flow to injured tissues.	Relieves pain, reduces inflammation
Heat/Thermotherapy	Heat in the form of hot compresses, heat lamps, or heating pads, causes blood vessels to dilate and increases blood flow to injury site.	Relieves pain, enhances healing by increased blood flow removing cell debris from damaged tissues and carrying healing nutrients to injury site
Ultrasound	High-frequency sound waves produce deep heat applied directly to injured area.	Stimulates blood flow to promote healing
Massage	Manual pressing, rubbing, and manipulating of muscles	Soothes tense muscles and promotes healing by increasing blood flow to injury site

Source: Institute of Arthritis and Musculoskeletal and Skin Diseases, "Sports Injuries," April 2009. www.niams.nih.gov.

Spinal Cord Injuries Are Often Untreatable

Most sports-related injuries can be treated successfully, enabling athletes to fully recover and, in many cases, return to their sport. But the same is not always true of spinal cord injuries, which can lead to permanent disability. A study published in 2010 by Frederick O. Mueller and Robert C. Cantu of the National Center for Catastrophic Sports Injury Research focused on spinal cord injuries among football players at all levels, and found that over a 34-year period 314 players were left paralyzed—and over 82 percent of these were high school age.

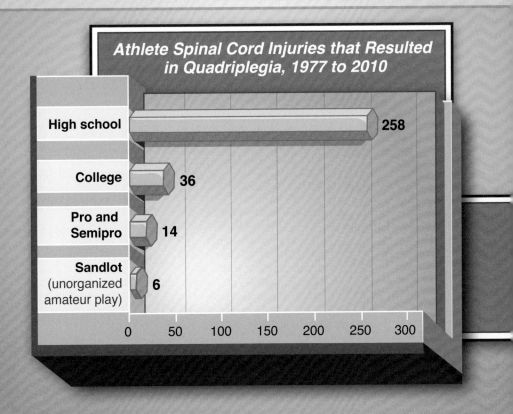

Source: Frederick O. Mueller and Robert C. Cantu, *Annual Survey of Catastrophic Football Injuries: 1977–2010.* www.unc.edu.

- Orthopedic surgeon Jonathan Cluett says that on rare occasions, an athlete who suffers from a severe groin pull may have a **muscle rupture** that requires surgery to reattach the torn ends of the muscle.

- According to the National Athletic Trainers' Association, only **42 percent** of high schools have access to a certified athletic trainer or physician during games and practices.

- According to James Harding, a dentist in Vail, Colorado, young athletes who have a tooth knocked out can expect over **$20,000** in lifetime dental costs associated with that one tooth.

- The STOP Sports Injuries campaign says that most ankle sprains can be treated with **bracing** and **physical therapy**, rather than surgery.

- Exercise physiologist Elizabeth Quinn says that if an athlete does not take a several-week break from activity after suffering a **stress fracture**, reinjury can occur and the stress fracture may never heal properly.

- According to Ron Courson, the director of sports medicine at the University of Georgia, unlike most sports injuries, no treatment or rehabilitation exercises exist for athletes who suffer from **concussions**; the only treatment is physical and mental rest.

- The NIAMS says that the vast majority of sports injuries **do not require surgery**.

How Can Sports Injuries Be Prevented?

"Sports medicine needs to evolve into a field that tries to prevent injuries instead of simply treating them."

—David Geier, an orthopedic surgeon and director of the Sports Medicine Program at the Medical University of South Carolina.

"Coaches, athletes, and parents must be aware of the possible injuries and follow the rules in place to prevent them. Serious injuries can be avoided if players avoid dangerous tactics or overly aggressive play."

—American Academy of Orthopaedic Surgeons, which engages in health policy and advocacy activities on behalf of patients and the orthopedic surgery profession.

Christopher Nowinski is one of the most prominent advocates for football reform in the United States—and he is someone who knows firsthand how hard life can be after a brain injury. A former football player for Harvard University, Nowinski was a professional wrestler until problems from repeated concussions forced him to retire at the age of 24. "I was left with an unreliable memory," he says, "daily throbbing headaches, depression, and even developed a dangerous sleepwalking habit."[50] Nowinski is now codirector of the Center for the Study of Traumatic Encephalopathy at Boston University School of Medicine. As the organization's name implies, its primary focus is on chronic traumatic encephalopathy (CTE), a degenerative brain disease that is directly

linked to repeated blows to the head. "In layman's term," says Nowinski, "hitting your head thousands of times appears to create a disease that slowly and quietly causes your brain cells to die."[51]

Preventive Measures Are Needed

On January 4, 2010, Nowinski testified before the US House of Representatives in a hearing about football-related head injuries. He emphasized the tragic nature of CTE and made it clear that the only way to stop the devastating disorder was through efforts that would keep it from happening in the first place. "We cannot diagnose it while someone is alive," he told the group. "We cannot treat it and we cannot cure it. Today, we can only prevent it, but to do this we have to dig deep and find the will, because this Friday night, in small towns across America, you can be sure we are creating it."[52]

In his closing remarks, Nowinski said that football needs to be re-evaluated at youth, high school, college, and professional levels, and that preventive measures are essential. "This is a unique opportunity to change the course of the lives of millions of young men and women," he said, "and to cut off a growing public health problem at the pass. . . . We are dealing with children, and we are dealing with a problem that can be significantly remedied quickly and cheaply tomorrow. We just have to decide if we have the will."[53]

Tougher Rules for Rough Sports

After years of being criticized for its lackadaisical attitude about head injuries among pro football players, the NFL has taken major steps toward better management of concussions. For instance, prior to 2009 the organization's policy was to send players back into the game as soon as visible symptoms of concussions subsided. But when faced with overwhelming evidence that numerous retired players were suffering from permanent brain damage, the league implemented more stringent rules. The impetus for these rule changes was a September 2009 study commissioned by the NFL, which showed that Alzheimer's disease or similar memory-related disorders were being diagnosed in former pro football players at 19 times the rate that was normal for adult males. The following December the NFL announced that it would require any player with signs of concussion to be removed from a game (or practice) and not be

allowed to return the same day. Another requirement was for players to be examined by a physician who specializes in recognizing and treating concussions.

In 2010 the NFL tightened its rules even further, announcing that it would impose stiff fines against players who make deliberate and/or violent hits, especially those that result in blows to the head. And as the 2011 football season approached, the NFL was continuing to explore efforts to reduce concussions among players. Researchers at the group's Southern Impact Research Center in Rockford, Tennessee, have been examining ways to install sensors (known as accelerometers) on football helmets. These are designed to measure the amount of head trauma players receive when they are hit.

> " After years of being criticized for its lackadaisical attitude about head injuries among pro football players, the NFL has taken major steps toward better management of concussions. "

If the experiment works as planned, the sensors would be installed in the helmets worn by a test sample of players in an actual game. Kevin Guskiewicz, director of sports-related brain injury research at the University of North Carolina and a member of the NFL's head, neck, and spine committee, explains: "The purpose is to find out in real time out on the field, as opposed to in a laboratory like we're doing here, what types of impacts players take."[54] Using this technology, the researchers hope to learn why some players sustain hard hits to the head and are unaffected, while others suffer concussions.

Because concussions are also an ongoing problem in pro hockey, the National Hockey League (NHL) has taken its own steps to reduce head injuries among players. After a series of meetings in March 2011, NHL commissioner Gary Bettman announced that the league would change its practice of evaluating players who have potentially sustained concussions. Under the new protocol, any player who exhibits concussion symptoms must be examined by the team physician in a quiet place, rather than being examined on the bench by an athletic trainer. The NHL will

also study ways to modify player equipment to make it safer and evaluate whether to toughen its rules about deliberate hits to the head.

Many health professionals are encouraged by these measures. But according to Canadian neurosurgeon Charles Tator, who founded the brain injury prevention agency ThinkFirst, the NHL needs to follow the lead of pro football. "I have great respect for the NFL's new attitude toward the head," he says. "I think they're ahead of the NHL in dealing with the concussion problem."[55]

Legislating Athlete Safety

When Zackery Lystedt was stricken with second-impact syndrome after a junior high school football game in 2006, his parents were focused entirely on his survival. After he began to recover from his injuries, he and his parents embarked on a quest: to do whatever they could to prevent other young athletes from suffering the same fate. They, along with attorney Richard H. Adler, who is president of the Brain Injury Association of Washington, created a piece of legislation called the Zackery Lystedt Law. It contains stringent return-to-play procedures for athletes under the age of 18, stating that they must be removed from a game or practice immediately if a concussion is suspected. Athletes will not be allowed to return to play without written medical clearance from a health-care provider who specializes in the evaluation and treatment of concussions. Also, athletes and their parents must be educated about the dangers of concussions each year and sign a document stating that they have been informed about and understand concussion dangers.

> As of September 2011, 32 states and the District of Columbia had passed student-athlete concussion laws, and similar legislation was pending in 10 states.

In May 2009 Washington became the first state to pass the Zachery Lystedt Law, with several other states passing similar laws over the following months. In May 2010 NFL commissioner Roger Goodell sent a letter to the governors of states that did not have such laws, urging them to pass legislation in order to better

protect young athletes. As of September 2011, 32 states and the District of Columbia had passed student-athlete concussion laws, and legislation was pending in 10 states. The thirty-second state to pass such a law was Delaware, whose legislation went into effect on August 30, 2011. After Governor Jack Markell signed the bill into law, he shared his thoughts about its importance:

> When you look at the data and the long-term effects of concussions—especially repeat concussions—it paints an alarming picture. Sports has gone beyond outdated adages about getting "dinged," "playing tough," and getting back into the game. Concussions can be serious, potentially life-changing injuries. We're stepping up and treating them with the seriousness they deserve.[56]

Crucial Protection

Sports injury specialists and neurosurgeons say that helmets should always be worn for any contact sport, as well as when participating in athletics such as biking and in-line skating. Other types of gear are also important, and according to the American Academy of Pediatrics (AAP), it is essential for all sports gear to fit properly. In addition to helmets (and depending on the sport), the group recommends pads for the neck, shoulders, elbows, chest, knees, and shins; mouthpieces; face guards; protective cups; and eyewear. The AAP adds, however, that athletes "should not assume that protective gear will protect them from performing more dangerous or risky activities."[57] Even when athletes are suited up in protective gear, getting hurt is still a possibility.

Most helmets, for example, are designed to protect against skull fractures but not concussions, and this has been a concern of health officials and sports medicine specialists for years. To inves-

> " Most helmets, for example, are designed to protect against skull fractures but not concussions, and this has been a concern of health officials and sports medicine specialists for years. "

tigate helmet safety, reporters from the *New York Times* interviewed experts and evaluated industry data, and then published the findings in an October 20, 2010, article. The research revealed that over 100,000 child athletes are wearing helmets that are too old to provide adequate protection, and an estimated half million others are wearing potentially unsafe helmets. *Times* reporter Alan Schwartz writes: "Helmets both new and used are not—and have never been— formally tested against the forces believed to cause concussions. The industry, which receives no governmental or other independent oversight, requires helmets for players of all ages to withstand only the extremely high-level force that would otherwise fracture skulls."[58]

Several manufacturers, including Ridell, Schutt, and Xenith, have developed helmets that are designed to reduce the risk of concussion by being lined with materials other than the traditional foam. The Xenith football helmet, for instance, is lined with 18 tiny shock absorbers that work like automobile airbags and inflate when the athlete sustains a blow to the head. These helmets were put to the test at Buckingham Browne & Nichols high school in Cambridge, Massachusetts. Players say that they can definitely tell the difference in how they feel when they get hit. John Papas, the school's football coach, says that with the new helmets, concussions dropped significantly from the prior year. "It was the best thing we've ever done,"[59] says Papas.

> When Wes Leonard collapsed on the basketball court, the only defibrillator the school owned was in a different building. His parents cannot help wondering if his life could have been saved if the machine had been available.

A Quest to Save Young Lives

After their son died from sudden cardiac arrest in March 2011, Jocelyn and Gary Leonard felt compelled to channel their grief into something that would benefit young athletes. So they formed the Wes Leonard Heart Team, a foundation whose mission is to prevent other athletes

from succumbing to sudden cardiac arrest. The group's focus is to raise public awareness and to get a law passed in Michigan that would require all schools to have automatic external defibrillators (AEDs) at every athletic practice and sporting event. An AED is a small, lightweight device that is used to assess a person's heart rhythm, and if necessary, it can administer an electric shock to restore a normal rhythm. When Wes Leonard collapsed on the basketball court, the only defibrillator the school owned was in a different building. His parents cannot help wondering if his life could have been saved if the machine had been available.

As of August 2011 the Wes Leonard Heart Team had raised $40,000 to buy defibrillators for schools. The group had handed out thousands of postcards with information about sudden cardiac arrest and had trained approximately 50 people at Fennville High School to use the defibrillators and to perform cardiopulmonary resuscitation. The Leonards met with a state senator who planned to introduce a bill that would require AEDs in all Michigan schools. "We have to look out for all kids," says Jocelyn Leonard. "All kids deserve one more game. My kid deserved one more game. We can honor him by changing the law to make more kids safe."[60]

The Ultimate Goal

Although most sports injuries can be treated effectively, prevention is the ultimate goal. Says Christine MacDonell, who is the managing director of medical rehabilitation with the accrediting firm CARF International: "Sports medicine offers many tools to help all athletes whether Olympians, professionals, or weekend warriors recover from sports injuries; however, the best way to deal with an injury is not to have one at all."[61] Prevention measures have been shown to vastly reduce sports injuries, from higher-quality equipment and more stringent rules to legislation designed to better protect athletes. These and other future efforts will undoubtedly help keep athletes of all ages safer than they are today.

How Can Sports Injuries Be Prevented?

66 **Whether they are pursuing gold medals or leisure, those who participate in physical activity require both proper preventive training and proper health-care; they will benefit greatly from experts who can deliver these.** 99

—Paul Comfort and Earle Abrahamson, eds., *Sports Rehabilitation and Injury Prevention*. West Sussex, UK: Wiley-Blackwell, 2010.

Comfort and Abrahamson are sports medicine specialists from the United Kingdom.

66 **The public health crisis is already here and we cannot afford to wait any longer to make changes to the way we play sports at high risk of head trauma. Blows to the head need to be minimized through rule and technique changes, especially in those sports such as football that are being played in a far different manner than originally conceived.** 99

—Robert C. Cantu, testimony to the US House Judiciary Committee, October 28, 2009. http://judiciary.house.gov.

Cantu is a Boston neurosurgeon and noted expert on sports-related concussions who is cofounder of both the Sports Legacy Institute and the Center for the Study of Traumatic Encephalopathy at Boston University School of Medicine.

* Editor's Note: While the definition of a primary source can be narrowly or broadly defined, for the purposes of Compact Research, a primary source consists of: 1) results of original research presented by an organization or researcher; 2) eyewitness accounts of events, personal experience, or work experience; 3) first-person editorials offering pundits' opinions; 4) government officials presenting political plans and/or policies; 5) representatives of organizations presenting testimony or policy.

❝If we are to encourage young people to be healthy athletes who embrace ideas like teamwork and doing their best, then this Congress must do everything it can to protect them as they participate in sports. That is what we call 'fair play.'❞

—Bill Pascrell, testimony to the US House Judiciary Committee, October 28, 2009. http://judiciary.house.gov.

Pascrell is a US representative from New Jersey and cochair of the Congressional Brain Injury Task Force.

❝Prevention is better than cure. To prevent sports injuries, the first step is to ascertain whether a person choosing sports is fit to take it.❞

—John Ebnezar, *Textbook of Orthopedics*. New Delhi: Jaypee Brothers Medical, 2010.

Ebnezar is an orthopedic surgeon from Karnataka, India.

❝There is a strong and growing scientific basis to support appropriate prevention, identification, detection, and response for sports related concussions.❞

—Vikas Kapil, "Protecting School-Age Athletes from Sports-Related Concussion Injury," CDC congressional testimony, September 8, 2010. www.cdc.gov.

Kapil is a physician who serves as the associate director for science in the Division of Injury Response at the National Center for Injury Prevention and Control.

❝Heat-related illnesses are 100% preventable. That's right—it is the one thing athletic trainers and other medical professionals come across that can be stopped before it starts.❞

—BJ Maack, "If You Can't Take the Heat—Part II," *STOP Sports Injuries* (blog), August 10, 2011. www.stopsportsinjuries.org.

Maack is a certified athletic trainer with the Arkansas Sports Performance Center.

❝Parents play a large role in injury prevention. First, they must be careful not to encourage their children to advance to higher levels of training at an unsafe rate.❞

—American Orthopaedic Society for Sports Medicine, "Dance Injuries," *AOSSM Sports Tips*, 2009. www.sportsmed.org.

Composed of over 3,000 physicians and other health professionals, the society serves as a forum for education and research.

❝Although collisions with cars or other vehicles are likely to be the most serious, even a low-speed fall on a bicycle path can be dangerous. For kids and adults alike, wearing a bicycle helmet is the most effective way to prevent a life-threatening head injury.❞

—Mayo Clinic, "Fitness: Bicycle Helmet Do's and Don'ts," May 1, 2010. www.mayoclinic.com.

The Mayo Clinic is a world-renowned medical facility headquartered in Rochester, Minnesota.

❝In conditions of extreme heat or humidity when children or adolescents can no longer maintain thermal balance, safety should be the priority, and outdoor contests and practice sessions should be canceled or rescheduled to cooler times.❞

—AAP, "Policy Statement: Climatic Heat Stress and Exercising Children and Adolescents," *Pediatrics*, August 8, 2011. http://pediatrics.aappublications.org.

The AAP is composed of 60,000 physicians who specialize in pediatric medicine.

❝Surveillance studies of mouthguard users and nonusers have consistently shown that mouthguards offer significant protection against sports-related injuries to the teeth and soft tissues.❞

—American Dental Association, "Statement on Athletic Mouthguards," February 2009. www.ada.org.

Composed of over 157,000 members, the American Dental Association is the oldest and largest national dental society in the world.

How Can Sports Injuries Be Prevented?

- According to the CDC, over **50 percent** of all sports injuries among children and teenagers are preventable.

- The American Dental Association estimates that mandatory use of **athletic mouth guards** prevents about 200,000 injuries each year in high school and college football.

- The American Association of Neurological Surgeons says that children whose helmets fit poorly are twice as likely to sustain a **head injury** in a bicycle crash as those whose helmets fit properly.

- According to data from the National Ski Areas Association, **48 percent** of US skiers and snowboarders wore helmets during the 2008–2009 season, up from the 2002–2003 season, when **25 percent** wore helmets.

- The National Athletic Trainers' Association says that even the very best helmets cannot prevent an athlete from sustaining a **concussion**, as they are designed only to prevent **skull fractures**.

- According to the STOP Sports Injuries campaign, overuse injuries can often be prevented if an athlete does not increase his or her training program or activity more than **10 percent** per week.

- A 2011 study by researchers from the University of Wisconsin found that high school basketball players who wore **lace-up ankle braces** had a significantly lower rate of ankle injuries than those who did not wear the braces.

Preventing Repeat Concussions

Research shows that young people who sustain a second concussion before recovering from the first have an increased risk of long-term neurological effects. These findings have led to efforts to reduce the risk of concussion for school-age athletes. In a May 2010 survey of parents of school athletes age 12 to 17, respondents voiced strong support for school-based efforts to guard against repeat concussions. In the survey, conducted for the University of Michigan C.S. Mott Children's Hospital, a majority of parents voiced support for policies such as requiring clearance from a doctor before an athlete can return to play after a concussion.

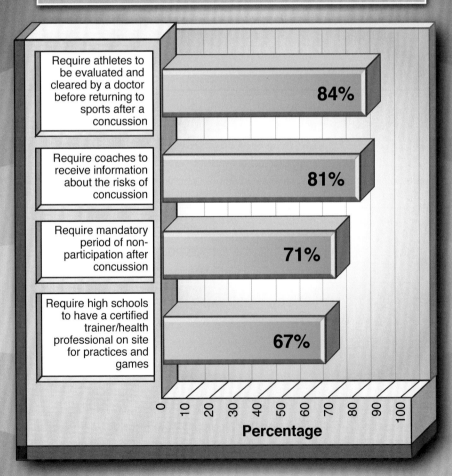

Percentage of Parents Who Say Schools Should . . .

- Require athletes to be evaluated and cleared by a doctor before returning to sports after a concussion — **84%**
- Require coaches to receive information about the risks of concussion — **81%**
- Require mandatory period of non-participation after concussion — **71%**
- Require high schools to have a certified trainer/health professional on site for practices and games — **67%**

Percentage

Source: C.S. Mott Children's Hospital, "Concussions in School Sports: Parents Ill-Prepared for Role in Reducing Kids' Risks," *National Poll on Children's Health*, June 14, 2010. www.med.umich.edu.

Laws to Protect Young Athletes

In May 2009 Washington became the first state to pass legislation focused on preventing concussions among young athletes and specifying what must happen if an athlete does sustain a concussion. As of September 1, 2011, 32 states and the District of Columbia had passed similar legislation, and laws were pending in 10 other states.

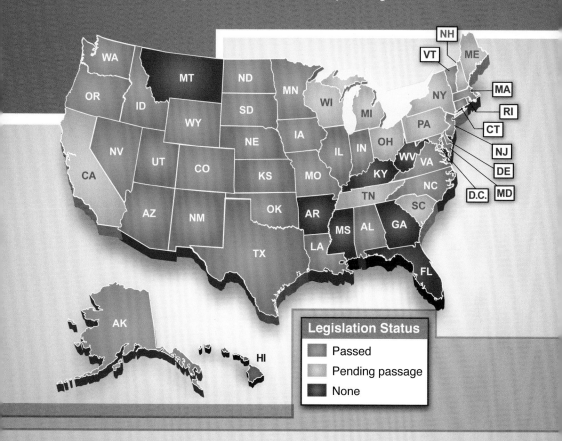

Source: Bryan Toporek, "Delaware Rings in School Year with New Concussion Law," *Education Week* blog, September 1, 2011. http://blogs.edweek.org.

- According to Ron Courson, the director of sports medicine at the University of Georgia, **concussion prevention efforts** must encompass safer techniques, procedure changes, more protective equipment, and proper enforcement of rules.

Heading Off Football Injuries

Health officials and sports medicine specialists emphasize that most sports injuries are preventable. Because football is such a popular sport—and one that often involves injuries—the American Orthopaedic Society for Sports Medicine and the American Academy of Orthopaedic Surgeons have developed strategies to help players avoid injury.

Prevention Strategies for Football Players

Have a preseason health and wellness evaluation to determine ability to participate.
Warm up properly with low-impact exercises such as walking that gradually increase heart rate.
Consistently incorporate strength training and stretching. A good stretch involves not going beyond the point of resistance and holding for 10 to 12 seconds.
Drink plenty of water to remain hydrated, minimize cramps, and maintain health.
Play multiple positions and/or sports during the offseason to minimize overuse injuries.
Wear properly fitted protective equipment such as a helmet, pads, shoes, and mouth guard. Do not modify equipment.
Tackle with the head up and do not lead with the helmet.
Cool down properly to lower heart rate gradually with exercises such as light jogging.
Do not play through the pain. Players should speak with an orthopaedic surgeon who specializes in sports medicine or an athletic trainer to discuss any concerns about possible injury.

Source: American Academy of Orthopaedic Surgeons, "Return of Football Season Brings Attention to High Injury Rates and Need for Prevention," September 8, 2010. www.aaos.org.

- The Children's Memorial Hospital in Chicago says that female athletes who participate in the facility's **Knee Injury Prevention Program (KIPP)** are up to nine times less likely to sustain a severe knee injury while playing sports.

Key People and Advocacy Groups

American National Standards Institute: An organization that establishes standards for products, services, systems, and personnel in the United States, including certifying protective equipment used in sports activities.

Robert C. Cantu: A Boston neurosurgeon and noted expert on sports-related concussions who is cofounder of both the Sports Legacy Institute and the Center for the Study of Traumatic Encephalopathy at Boston University School of Medicine.

James Garrick: A physician known as a sports medicine pioneer, Garrick founded the first academic sports medicine program in the United States during the 1960s in Vail, Colorado.

Roger Goodell: Commissioner of the NFL since 2006, Goodell was sharply criticized for the league's neglect in its management of active and retired players with brain injuries and was subsequently instrumental in getting tougher laws passed to guard against concussions.

Creighton J. Hale: A scientist and inventor who developed several types of baseball and softball safety equipment for youth players, including the double earflap batter's helmet, catcher's helmet, chest protector with throat guard, and the nonwood baseball bat.

Stephen D. Keener: The president and CEO of Little League Baseball, Keener has been instrumental in implementing safety enhancements for youth players.

Zackery Lystedt: A teenager from Washington who was left permanently disabled from second-impact syndrome in 2006 and whose work to protect other young athletes from concussions led to the creation of the Zackery Lystedt Law.

National Center for Sports Safety (NCSS): An organization that promotes the importance of injury prevention and safety in youth sports and seeks to decrease the number and/or severity of injuries through education and research.

National Collegiate Athletic Association (NCAA): Represents and oversees 23 collegiate sports, provides support to its members, enforces NCAA bylaws, and communicates with the public.

National Institute of Arthritis and Musculoskeletal and Skin Diseases: An organization that supports research into the causes, treatment, and prevention of arthritis and diseases of the musculoskeletal system and skin.

Christopher Nowinski: Codirector of the Center for the Study of Traumatic Encephalopathy at Boston University School of Medicine, the author of *Head Games: Football's Concussion Crisis*, and one of the country's most prominent advocates for football reform.

Linda Sánchez: A congresswoman from California who has been an outspoken critic of the NFL for its handling of players' concussions, comparing the league's stance on the problem with tobacco companies' denial that smoking causes cancer.

Sports Legacy Institute (SLI): An organization that seeks to solve the concussion crisis in sports and the military through medical research, treatment, education, and prevention.

Sports Trauma Overuse and Prevention (STOP): An outreach program created by the American Orthopaedic Society for Sports Medicine that educates the public about the importance of sports safety, specifically related to overuse and trauma injuries.

Chronology

1905
After the deaths of 18 college football players in one season, US president Theodore Roosevelt summons sports leaders from Harvard, Princeton, and Yale to the White House for a summit on football safety reform.

1979
The NHL makes helmets mandatory for all new players signing an NHL contract.

1971
Batting helmets become mandatory for all Major League Baseball players.

1939
The John T. Riddell Company of Chicago introduces the first hard plastic football helmet, designed to be more protective than the soft leather helmets in use at the time.

1943
The NFL makes it mandatory for players to wear protective headgear.

1900   1940   1980

1930
After having his nose broken by a flying puck, Montreal Maroons hockey player Clint Benedict becomes the first goaltender to wear a mask in an NHL game.

1952
The Pittsburgh Pirates become the first major league baseball team to permanently adopt batting helmets for all players.

1969
To address the prevalence of sports-related injuries and deaths, the National Operating Committee on Standards in Athletic Equipment is formed and is charged with commissioning research on injury reduction.

1906
The Intercollegiate Athletic Association of the United States is founded to reform college football rules; the group's responsibilities later expand to include all intercollegiate sports and its name is changed to the NCAA.

1973
The National Operating Committee on Standards in Athletic Equipment publishes the first test standard for football helmets in the United States.

1984

In a published paper, neurosurgeons Richard L. Saunders and Robert E. Harbaugh coin the term "second-impact syndrome" to describe the catastrophic brain injury that can occur after an athlete who has had a concussion sustains a second blow to the head.

2010

The youth football organization Pop Warner establishes a rule that any athlete who has sustained a head injury must obtain a note from a licensed medical professional who is trained in concussion management before returning to play.

2000

A study of nearly 1,100 former pro football players finds that over 60 percent suffered at least one concussion during their careers and 26 percent had three or more concussions.

2007

Little League Baseball institutes a rule that limits the number of pitches that can be thrown in a day, as well as the amount of rest required, based on the age of the pitcher.

1980

2000

2010

1996

After completing a comprehensive youth baseball safety study, the US Consumer Product Safety Commission concludes that safety equipment could reduce injuries in children's baseball by 36 percent.

2005

A University of North Carolina study finds that nearly 18 percent of retired NFL players who had at least one concussion during their careers suffer from permanent thinking or memory impairment.

2009

Washington becomes the first state to pass legislation mandating that athletes under the age of 18 who have suffered a concussion cannot return to play without written permission from a certified medical professional. Later the same year, the NFL imposes its own rules about when players should be allowed to return to games or practices after head injuries.

2011

Pro football player Joe Thomas and six former players file a federal class-action suit against the NFL, alleging that the league trained players to hit with their heads, failed to provide concussion treatment, and attempted to conceal links between football and brain injuries for decades.

Related Organizations

American Academy of Orthopaedic Surgeons (AAOS)

6300 N. River Rd.
Rosemont, IL 60018-4262
phone: (847) 823-7186 • fax: (847) 823-8125
e-mail: pemr@aaos.org • website: www.aaos.org

The AAOS engages in health policy and advocacy activities on behalf of patients and the orthopedic surgery profession. Its website offers news articles, press releases, and a search engine that produces a wide variety of articles about sports injuries.

American Orthopaedic Society for Sports Medicine (AOSSM)

6300 N. River Rd., Suite 500
Rosemont, IL 60018
phone: (847) 292-4900; toll-free: (877) 321-3500 • fax: (847) 292-4905
e-mail: info@aossm.org • website: www.sportsmed.org

Composed of over 3,000 physicians and other health professionals, the AOSSM serves as a forum for education and research. Its website offers the *In Motion* newsletter, podcasts, news releases, and a link to the organization's Sports Trauma Overuse and Prevention (STOP) campaign.

Brain Injury Association of America (BIAA)

1608 Spring Hill Rd., Suite 110
Vienna, VA 22182
phone: (703) 761-0750 • fax: (703) 761-0755
e-mail: info@biausa.org • website: www.biausa.org

The BIAA is the oldest and largest brain injury advocacy organization in the United States. Its website offers news releases, *The Challenge!* quarterly newsletter, a section with detailed information about brain injuries, and a fact sheet about sports-related concussions.

National Alliance for Youth Sports (NAYS)

2050 Vista Pkwy.
West Palm Beach, FL 33411
phone: (561) 684-1141; toll-free: (800) 729-2057 • fax: (561) 684-2546
e-mail: nays@nays.org • website: www.nays.org

The NAYS seeks to make sports safe, fun, and healthy for all children. Its website offers archived news articles, youth sports resources, the *National Standards for Youth Sports* publication, and a link to the group's Facebook page.

National Athletic Trainers' Association (NATA)

2952 Stemmons Fwy. #200
Dallas, TX 75247
phone: (214) 637-6282 • fax: (214) 637-2206
e-mail: info@nata.org • website: www.nata.org

With over 35,000 members worldwide, the NATA is a professional membership association for certified athletic trainers and others who support the athletic training profession. Its website offers information about health issues, athletic trainer terminology, facts about athletic trainers, news releases, and links to articles about concussions in sports.

National Center for Sports Safety (NCSS)

2316 First Ave. S.
Birmingham, AL 35233
phone: (205) 329-7535; toll-free: (866) 508-6277 • fax: (205) 329-7526
e-mail: info@sportssafety.org • website: www.sportssafety.org

The NCSS promotes the importance of injury prevention and safety in youth sports and seeks to decrease the number and/or severity of injuries through education and research. Its website features a group of sports injury facts, news articles, an online forum, and an "Ask the Expert" section that allows people to find answers to their questions about sports injuries.

National Collegiate Athletic Association (NCAA)

700 W. Washington St.
PO Box 6222
Indianapolis, IN 46206-6222
phone: (317) 917-6222 • fax: (317) 917-6888
website: www.ncaa.org

Representing 23 college sports, the NCAA provides support to its members, interprets legislation, enforces NCAA bylaws, and communicates with the public. Its website features news releases, a "Key Issues" section, information on concussion prevention and treatment, and a search engine that produces numerous articles about sports injuries.

National Institute of Arthritis and Musculoskeletal and Skin Diseases (NIAMS)

1 AMS Cir.
Bethesda, MD 20892-3675
phone: (301) 495-4484; toll-free: (877) 226-4267 • fax: (301) 718-6366
e-mail: NIAMSinfo@mail.nih.gov • website: www.niams.nih.gov

An agency of the National Institutes of Health, the NIAMS supports research into the causes, treatment, and prevention of illnesses and injuries that affect bones, joints, muscles, and skin. Its website offers a health information index, news releases, research updates, and a search engine that produces numerous articles about sports injuries.

Safe Kids USA

1301 Pennsylvania Ave. NW, Suite 1000
Washington, DC 20004-1707
phone: (202) 662-0600 • fax: (202) 393-2072
e-mail: info@safekids.org • website: www.safekids.org

In an effort to prevent unintentional childhood injury, Safe Kids USA educates families and advocates for better laws to help keep children safe and healthy. Its website offers numerous articles and fact sheets about sports injuries, as well as research reports, position statements, brochures, and a link to the *Safe Kids Blog*.

Sports Legacy Institute (SLI)

PO Box 181225
Boston, MA 02118
phone: (617) 951-3799 • fax: (617) 951-1354
e-mail: info@sportslegacy.org • website: www.sportslegacy.org

The SLI seeks to solve the concussion crisis in sports and the military through medical research, treatment, education, and prevention. Its website offers news releases, educational information about concussions and long-term effects, archived newsletters, a "7 Steps for Brain Safety" guideline sheet for youth sports, and other publications.

Sports Trauma Overuse and Prevention (STOP)

6300 N. River Rd., Suite 500
Rosemont, IL 60018
phone: (847) 655-8660
e-mail: info@stopsportsinjuries.org • website: www.stopsportsinjuries.org

STOP is an outreach program that educates the public about the importance of sports safety, specifically related to overuse and trauma injuries. A wealth of information can be found on the website, including injury prevention booklets for all types of sports, an informative publication about concussions, videos, podcasts, and links to news articles.

US Sports Academy

One Academy Dr.
Daphne, AL 36526
phone: (251) 626-3303; toll-free: (800) 223-2668
e-mail: info@ussa.edu • website: www.ussa.edu

The US Sports Academy is the largest sports university in the world. Its website offers current news and events, the *Sport Digest* blog, the *Sport Journal* monthly publication, and a search engine that produces numerous articles related to sports injuries.

For Further Research

Books

Michael Hutson and Cathy Speed, eds., *Sports Injuries*. New York: Oxford University Press, 2011.

Dorling Kindersley, *Everyday Sports Injuries*. New York: DK, 2010.

Hal Marcovitz, *Sports Injuries*. Farmington Hills, MI: Lucent, 2010.

William P. Meehan, *Kids, Sports, and Concussions*. Santa Barbara, CA: Praeger, 2011.

Christopher M. Norris, *Managing Sports Injuries: A Guide for Students and Clinicians*. Edinburgh, NY: Churchill Livingstone/Elsevier, 2011.

Clifford D. Stark with Elizabeth Shimer Bowers, *Living with Sports Injuries*. New York: Facts On File, 2010.

Periodicals

Buzz Bissinger, "Texas Football and the Price of Paralysis," *Time*, January 27, 2010.

Nichole Buswell, "Flying High: Grinds and Space Walks. Backflips and Front Flips. Landing a 180 on the Half-Pipe," *Current Health Teens*, a Weekly Reader publication, November 2010.

Brian Cazeneuve, "A Painful Lesson," *Sports Illustrated*, March 21, 2011.

Guy Falotico, "Heading Off Trouble: Concussions Can Be More than Just a Headache," *Current Health Teens*, a *Weekly Reader* publication, November 2010.

Kate Huvane Gamble, "A New Game Plan for Concussion," *Neurology Now*, February/March 2011.

Sean Gregory, "The Problem with Football: How to Make It Safer," *Time*, February 8, 2010.

Cathy Gulli, "Concussions: The Untold Story," *MacLean's*, May 30, 2011.

Gary Mihoces, "NFL to Broaden Enforcement of Facemasking Rule," *USA Today*, August 8, 2011.

Steve Rushin, "Name That Pain," *Sports Illustrated*, July 25, 2011.

Rachel Saslow, "Cold, Hard, and Fast: The Danger of Winter Olympics Sports," *Washington Post*, February 16, 2010.

Alan Schwarz, "As Injuries Rise, Scant Oversight of Helmet Safety," *New York Times*, October 20, 2010.

USA Today Special Newsletter Edition, "Hockey Injuries Rising Among Kids," February 2011.

Internet Sources

Caleb Daniloff, "Game Changers: How Dramatic Brain Discoveries Are Influencing America's Most Popular Sport," *Bostonia,* Boston University, Fall, 2010. www.bu.edu/bostonia/fall10/football.

Wayne Drehs, "Nathan Stiles Wanted to Keep Playing," ESPN.com, November 17, 2010. http://sports.espn.go.com/espn/otl/news/story?id=5818575.

National Institute of Arthritis and Musculoskeletal and Skin Diseases, "Sports Injuries," April 2009. www.niams.nih.gov/Health_Info/Sports_Injuries/default.asp#ra_7.

Nemours Foundation, "Dealing with Sports Injuries," TeensHealth, August 2010. http://kidshealth.org/teen/safety/first_aid/sports_injuries.html.

Stephanie Pappas, "Hard-Hitting Sports Hold Dangers for Teen Athletes," LiveScience, September 23, 2010. www.livescience.com/8650-hard-hitting-sports-hold-dangers-teen-athletes.html.

PBS *Frontline*, "Football High: Attention Players, Parents, Coaches," April 12, 2011. www.pbs.org/wgbh/pages/frontline/football-high/attention-players-parents-coaches.

ScienceDaily, "Pediatric Sports Injuries: The Silent Epidemic," March 12, 2010. www.sciencedaily.com/releases/2010/03/100310083441.htm.

Terry Zeigler, "Second Impact Syndrome," SportsMD, May 21, 2010. www.sportsmd.com/Articles/id/38/n/second_impact_syndrome.aspx.

Source Notes

Overview

1. Quoted in Wayne Drehs, "Nathan Stiles Wanted to Keep Playing," ESPN.com, November 17, 2010. http://sports.espn.go.com.
2. Sean Gregory, "The Problem with Football: How to Make It Safer," *Time*, January 28, 2010, p. 36.
3. Quoted in Matt Higgins, "Still Healing, but Back at X Games as Spectator," *New York Times*, January 27, 2011. www.nytimes.com.
4. Joseph Iero, "Chronic or Overuse Injuries in Sports," National Center for Sports Safety, 2011. www.sportssafety.org.
5. National Institute of Arthritis and Musculoskeletal and Skin Diseases, "Sports Injuries," April 2009. www.niams.nih.gov.
6. Florida Hospital Sports Medicine, "Burners/Stingers," 2011. www.thesportsmedicineteam.com.
7. Centers for Disease Control and Prevention, "Cole's Story," *Injury Center Connection Newsletter*, Spring/Summer 2011. www.cdc.gov.
8. Quoted in Cathy Gulli, "Concussions: The Untold Story," *MacLean's*, May 30, 2011, p. 56.
9. National Institute of Arthritis and Musculoskeletal and Skin Diseases, "Sports Injuries."
10. Daniel Evans, interviewed by Tim Polzer, "Baylor Health Care System: Proper Sports Injury Rehab," iHigh, March 22, 2011. www.ihigh.com.
11. Quoted in *Orthopaedic & Neurosurgery Specialists* (blog), "Keeping Summer Sports Fun and Injury Free," July 12, 2010. http://blog.onsmd.com.
12. Quoted in Gregory, "The Problem with Football," p. 36.

What Are Sports Injuries?

13. Quoted in Prameet Kumar, "Penn Cyclist Recovering After Injury," *Daily Pennsylvanian*, August 20, 2011. http://thedp.com.
14. Quoted in ESPN.com, "Luis Salazar Returns to Braves Camp," March 23, 2011. http://sports.espn.go.com.
15. Robert Donatelli, "Muscle Imbalance and Common Overuse Injuries," SportsMD, April 25, 2011. www.sportsmd.com.
16. Quoted in Matt LeCren, "DeBruler's Killer Career Not Over Yet," *Downers Grove (IL) Patch*, December 28, 2010. http://downersgrove.patch.com.
17. Quoted in LeCren, "DeBruler's Killer Career Not Over Yet."
18. Quoted in LeCren, "DeBruler's Killer Career Not Over Yet."
19. Quoted in Ellin Holohan, "Youth Sports Injuries Reaching Epidemic Levels, Experts Report," Medicine Net, December 7, 2010. www.medicinenet.com.
20. Quoted in Mike Celizic, "Lindsey Vonn Reveals Serious Injury to Shin," MSNBC.com, February 10, 2010. http://today.msnbc.msn.com.
21. American Association of Neurological Surgeons, "Sports-Related Head Injury," July 2010. www.aans.org.
22. Terry Zeigler, "Second Impact Syndrome," SportsMD, May 21, 2010. www.sportsmd.com.
23. Matt Rybaltowski, "Young Player Helps Turn Trauma into Action on Concussions," CBS Sports, February

14, 2010. www.cbssports.com.

24. Quoted in Lindsay Cohen, "'He's Looked Fear in the Face, and He's Won,'" KOMO News, June 11, 2011. www.komonews.com.

How Serious a Problem Are Injuries in Youth Sports?

25. Quoted in Mike Wagner and Todd Jones, "Kids' Play, Serious Pain," *Columbus (OH) Dispatch*, August 30, 2010. www.dispatch.com.

26. Quoted in Wagner and Jones, "Kids' Play, Serious Pain."

27. Quoted in Heidi Splete, "Concussion Rates Rising in Younger Athletes," American College of Emergency Physicians, October 2010. www.acep.org.

28. Quoted in Katie Moisse, "Concussion Leaves 14-Year-Old Basketball Player Amnesic, Left-Handed," ABC News, February 24, 2011. http://abcnews.go.com.

29. Quoted in American Academy of Orthopaedic Surgeons, "Pediatric Sports Injuries: The Silent Epidemic," March 10, 2010. www6.aaos.org.

30. Quoted in Lisa Weisenberger, "Limiting the Pitch Count for Young Athletes," *AAOS Now*, April 2011. www.aaos.org.

31. Quoted in Allyson Angle, "Former Alabama Baseball Player Changes Career Path After Tommy John Surgery," *Overuse Injuries* (blog), March 30, 2011. http://overuse.ua.edu.

32. Quoted in Angle, "Former Alabama Baseball Player Changes Career Path After Tommy John Surgery."

33. Quoted in Allyson Angle, "Youth Sports Overuse Injuries on the Rise, Preventable," *Anniston (AL) Star*, July 24, 2011. www.annistonstar.com.

34. Quoted in Melissa Dahl, "Flying Without a Net: Cheer Injuries on Rise," MSNBC.com, May 20, 2010. www.msnbc.msn.com.

35. Quoted in Matthew Stanmyre and Jackie Friedman, "Kids and Concussions: One of the Most Dangerous Sports of All—Cheerleading," *New Jersey Star-Ledger*, January 4, 2010. http://blog.nj.com.

36. Quoted in Sue Thoms, "Study Finds Student Athlete Sudden Cardiac Deaths like Fennville Star Wes Leonard Are as Rare as Deaths from Lightning," MLive, March 4, 2011. www.mlive.com.

37. Quoted in Sue Thoms, "'This Would Have Been His Year,' Wes Leonard's Mother Says as Football Season Begins," MLive, August 7, 2011. www.mlive.com.

How Are Sports Injuries Treated?

38. Quoted in Lynn Jolly, "Despite a Life-Changing Rugby Accident Inspirational Connor Is Confident He Can Conquer 96-Mile Walk," *Paisley Daily Express* Scotland, March 7, 2011. www.paisleydailyexpress.co.uk.

39. Quoted in Samantha Booth, "Teenager Told He'd Never Be Able to Move Again Set to Walk West Highland Way," *Daily Record* (UK), June 4, 2011. www.dailyrecord.co.uk.

40. Quoted in *Now Rugby*, "Docherty Strides to Victory," June 13, 2011. www.nowrugby.com.

41. National Institute of Arthritis and Musculoskeletal and Skin Diseases, "Sports Injuries."

42. Richard B. Frobell et al. "A Randomized Trial of Treatment for Acute Anterior Cruciate Ligament Tears," *New England Journal of Medicine*, July 22, 2010. www.nejm.org.

43. Quoted in Frank Deford, "For Young Athletes, ACL Surgery Could Portend Life of Pain," *Sports Illustrated*, January 19, 2011. http://sportsillustrated

.cnn.com.

44. American Orthopaedic Society for Sports Medicine, *Arthroscopy*, 2008. www.sportsmed.org.

45. National Institute of Arthritis and Musculoskeletal and Skin Diseases, "Sports Injuries."

46. Quoted in *Medical News Today*, "Arthroscopic Hip Surgery May Fully Restore Function in Athletes," July 20, 2010. www.medicalnewstoday.com.

47. Michael Stuart, "Concussions in Sports Should Be Watched For and Treated, Not Dismissed," Mayo Clinic *Medical Edge*, March 6, 2008. www.mayoclinic.org.

48. Quoted in Kate Huvane Gamble, "A New Game Plan for Concussion," *Neurology Now*, February/March 2011, p. 30.

49. Quoted in Teresa Chin, "Clinic Studying iPad App to Screen for Concussions," Cleveland Live, August 23, 2011. www.cleveland.com.

How Can Sports Injuries Be Prevented?

50. Christopher Nowinski, "Legal Issues Relating to Football Head Injuries," testimony to the US House Judiciary Committee, October 28, 2009. http://judiciary.house.gov.

51. Nowinski, "Legal Issues Relating to Football Head Injuries."

52. Nowinski, "Legal Issues Relating to Football Head Injuries."

53. Nowinski, "Legal Issues Relating to Football Head Injuries."

54. Quoted in Gary Mihoces, "Helmet Sensors Could Soon Measure NFL's Biggest Hits," *USA Today*, June 17, 2011. www.usatoday.com.

55. Quoted in Robert Cribb, "High-Tech Helmets Result of Search for Concussion-Proof Solution," *Toronto Star*, March 11, 2011. www.thestar.com.

56. Quoted in *Newark (DE) Post*, "Governor Signs Law to Protect Student Athletes from Concussions," August 30, 2011. www.newarkpostonline.com.

57. American Academy of Pediatrics, "2011 Sports Injury Prevention Tip Sheet," 2011. www.aap.org.

58. Alan Schwarz, "As Injuries Rise, Scant Oversight of Helmet Safety," *New York Times*, October 20, 2010. www.nytimes.com.

59. Quoted in WHDH News, "Helmet Developed in MA Prevents Football Concussions," November 15, 2010. www1.whdh.com.

60. Quoted in Sue Thoms, "Wes Leonard's Parents Work for Law Requiring Defibrillators in Schools, so All Kids Can Play 'One More Game,'" MLive, June 22, 2011. www.mlive.com.

61. Christine M. MacDonell, "Teamwork Between Patients and Therapists Is Central to Sports Medicine," *Newsweek*, February 2, 2010. www.newsweekshowcase.com.

List of Illustrations

Index

Note: Boldface page numbers indicate
illustrations.

About the Author

Peggy J. Parks holds a bachelor of science degree from Aquinas College in Grand Rapids, Michigan, where she graduated magna cum laude. An author who has written more than 100 educational books for children and young adults, Parks lives in Muskegon, Michigan, a town that she says inspires her writing because of its location on the shores of Lake Michigan.

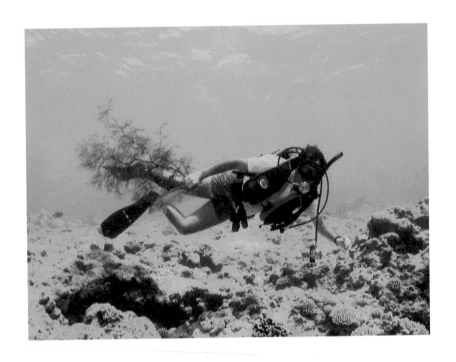

Shark teeth do not have roots like yours.
Their teeth often break or fall out.
Then new teeth move up from the
row behind.
They take the place of the lost teeth.

Sharks can lose thousands of teeth in
a lifetime.
Divers find many on the ocean floor.
Sailors used to shave with them!

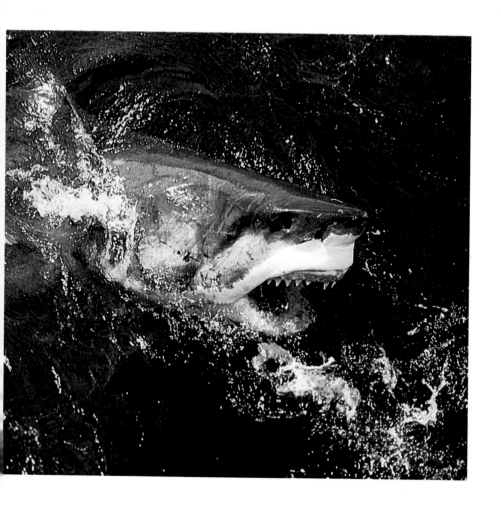

Sharks have teeth that are fit for what
they eat.

- Curved teeth are for biting.
- Pointed teeth are for catching
  small fish.
- Flat teeth are for crushing
  shellfish.

Shark teeth are not in one row like yours.
Sharks have as many as 20 rows
of teeth.
The rows are behind each other.

When a shark is ready to eat, it lifts
its snout.
This pushes the shark's mouth out
in front.
It also bares its teeth.

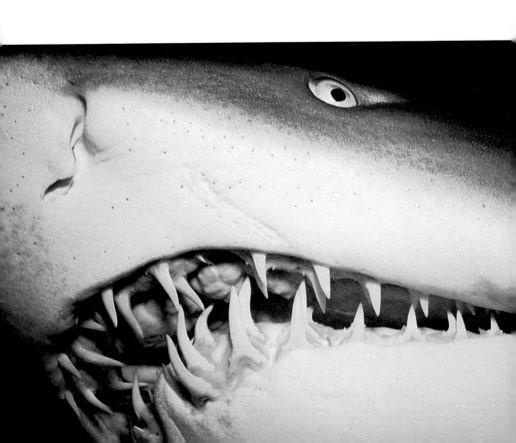

CHAPTER THREE

Hundreds of Teeth

Sharks have lots of teeth.

Some have hundreds.

A few have thousands.

Imagine brushing that many teeth!

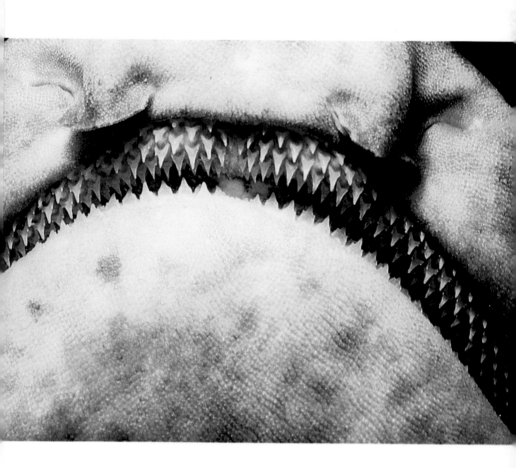

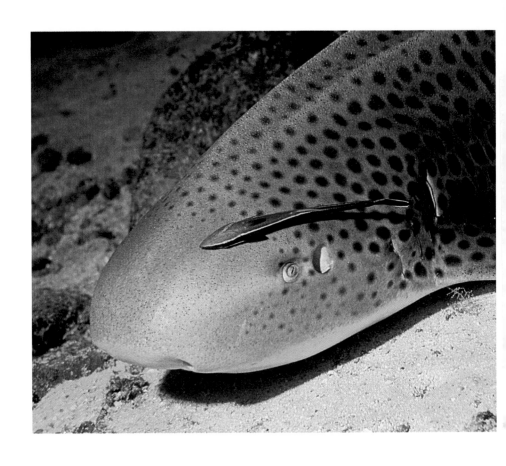

The other friend is the remora.

Remoras hitch rides on sharks.

They also eat shellfish that dig into the
sharks' skin.

No wonder sharks don't seem to mind
remoras tagging along.

Sharks often swim with two types of trusty friends.

One is the pilot fish.

Pilot fish seem to lead the sharks.

But all they do is catch food that the sharks drop.

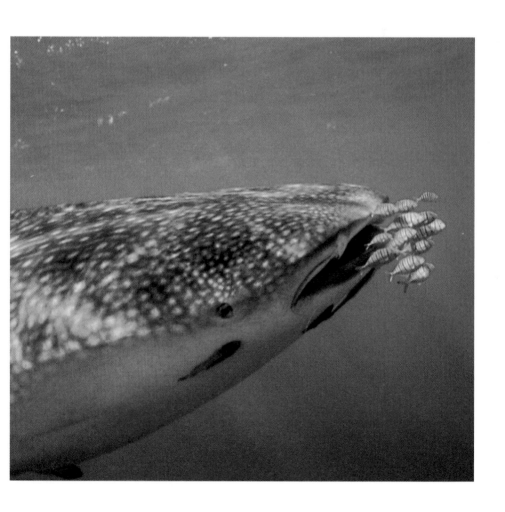

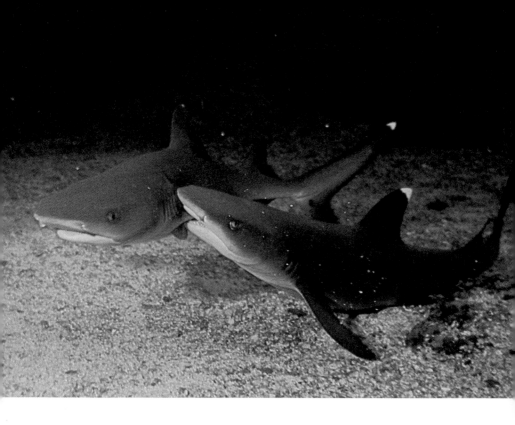

A shark twists and turns as it swims.
That's because it doesn't have a bone
in its body!
A shark's skeleton is made of cartilage
(say "CAR-ti-luj").
And cartilage bends easily.

Your nose has cartilage.
See how easily you can twist and
turn it.

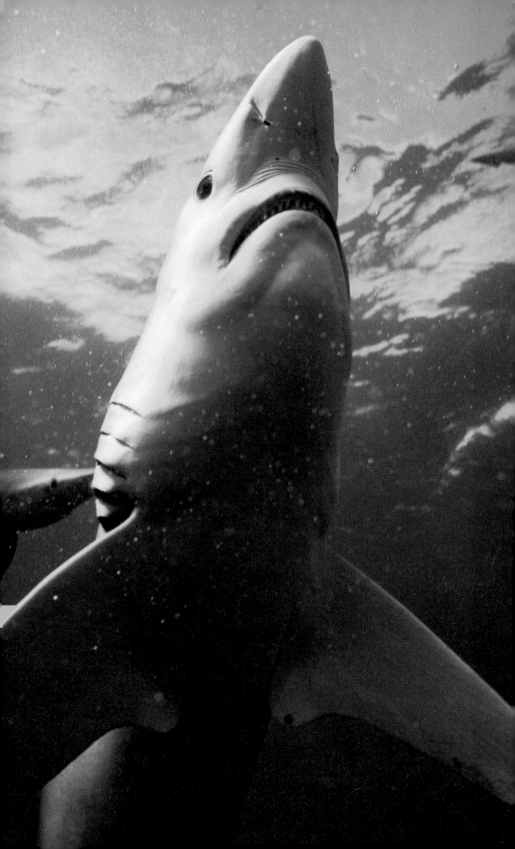

Now you know.

Sharks

- are mighty hunters,
- are powerful swimmers,
- have lots of teeth,
- give birth to pups,
- live almost everywhere,
- and come in all sizes and shapes.

They're really amazing!

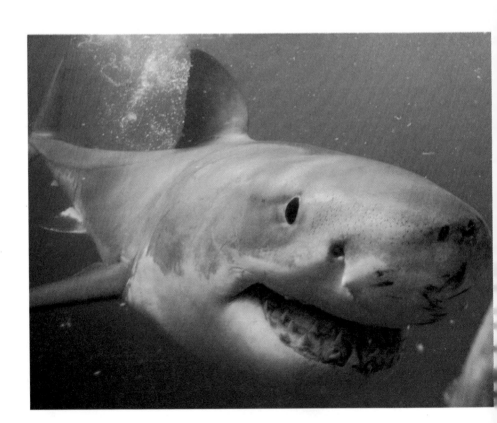

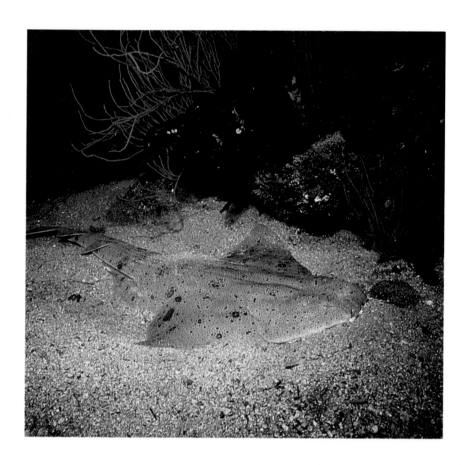

The **angel shark** is no angel.
It hides in reefs or caves under the
water.
Or it digs its body into the sand.
Nearby shellfish have to be careful.
The angel shark is always ready
to pounce.

It's easy to mistake the **carpet shark** for a rug.
It lays still on the ocean bottom.
Fringes around its snout make it look messy.
But let a fish swim by.
The carpet shark whips around and grabs it!

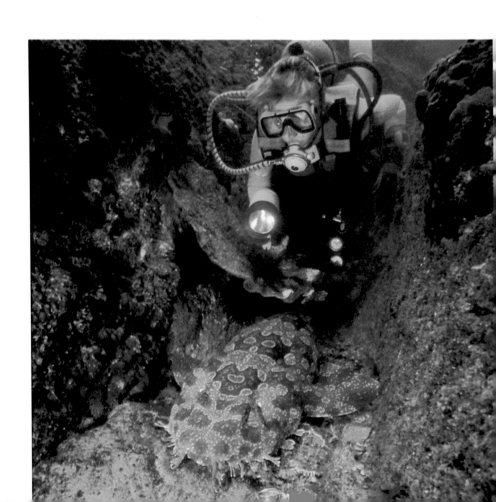

The **hammerhead shark** looks odd,
to say the least.
It has a thick bar across the front of
its head.
And its eyes are at the ends of the bar.
No one is sure why.

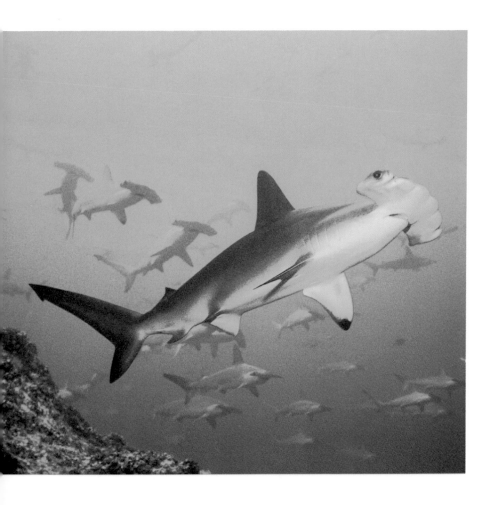

The biggest shark is the **whale shark**.
It can be as long and heavy as a
tractor trailer!
Sometimes the whale shark stands
upright in the water.
It bobs up and down, swallowing whole
schools of small fish.

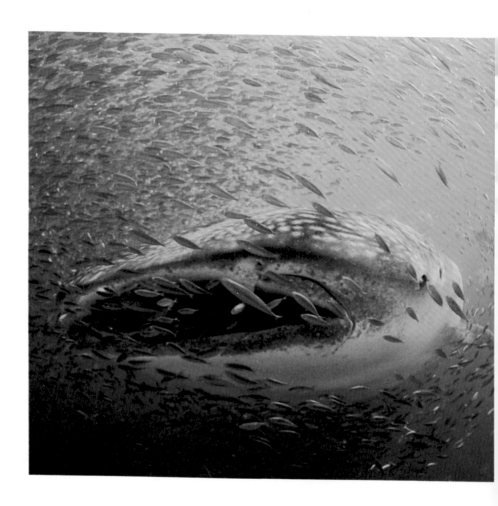

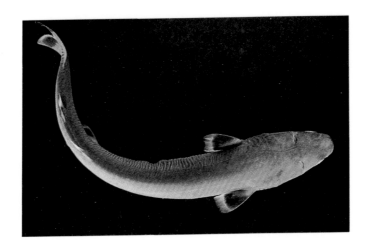

One of the smallest sharks is the **dwarf shark**.

It is only about six inches long.

You could hold one in your hand.

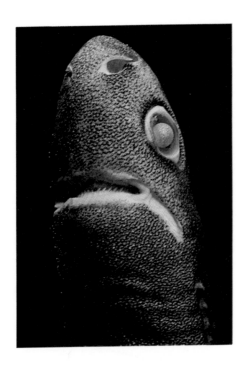

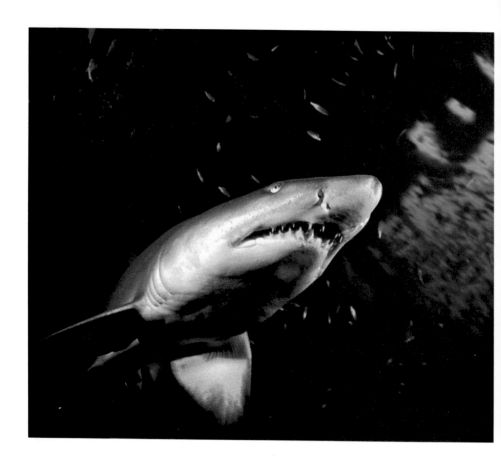

Some people call the **tiger shark**
a "swimming garbage can."
It will eat just about anything.
A fisherman once caught a tiger shark.
In its belly he found

- nine shoes,
- a belt,
- and a pair of pants!

The **blue shark** is easy to spot.
It lives in the deepest part of the
ocean.
Yet it swims near the surface.
Its fins stick up out of the water.
Blues often swim together in
large groups.

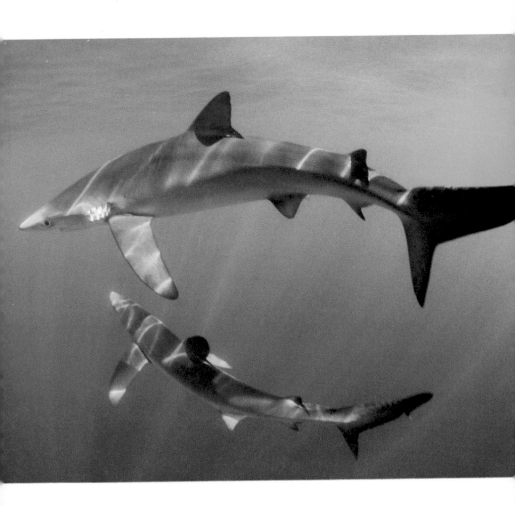

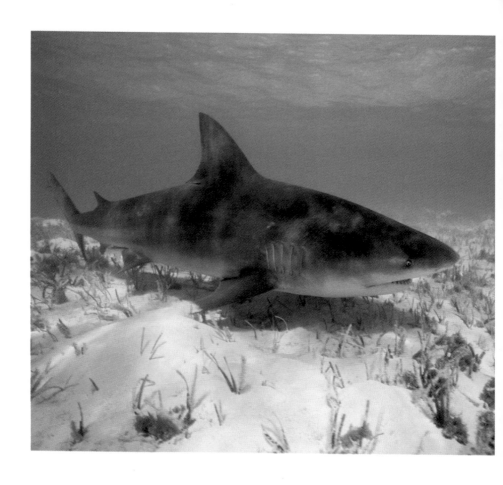

The **bull shark** is mostly found in shallow water.
Sometimes it swims into rivers or lakes.
A short snout and stout body make it look like a bull.
That's how it got its name.

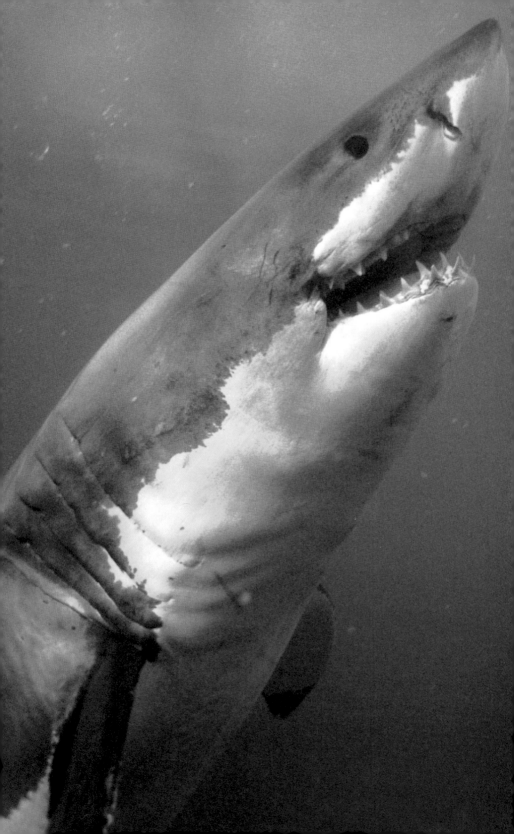

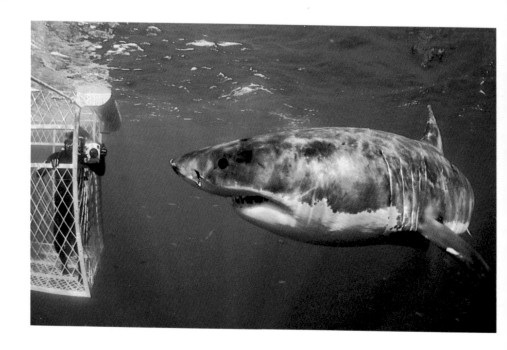

The **great white shark** swims mainly
in deep, cold seas.
Its underside is white.
But its back is dark.
This makes the great white hard to see.

- From below, the shark looks like
  the sky.
- From above, the shark looks like
  the water.

Large animals, such as sea lions, fall
prey to the great white shark.

CHAPTER FIVE

Curious Creatures

Sharks live all over the world.

- They live in deep water and shallow water.
- They live in cold water and warm water.
- Some even live in rivers and lakes.

Nearly everyone is afraid of sharks.
Yet most rarely harm us.

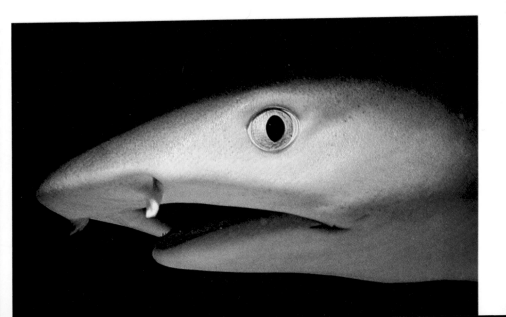

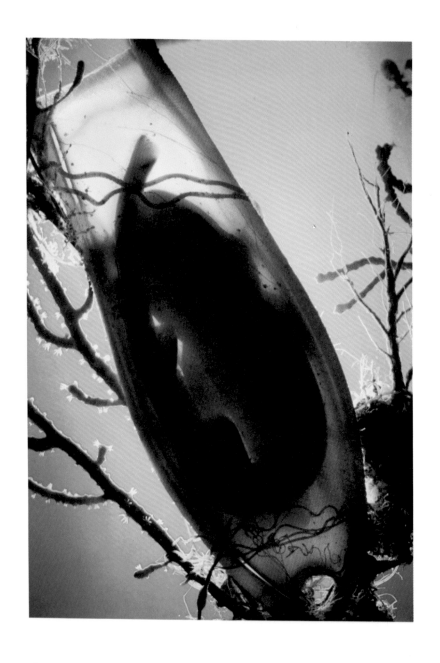

Sometimes egg cases wash ashore.
People find them on the beach.
They call the cases "mermaids' purses."

Some mother sharks lay eggs outside their bodies.
The eggs are in cases.
The cases fall to the bottom of the sea.

The pup grows inside the egg case.
When it hatches, the pup swims out —
and away!

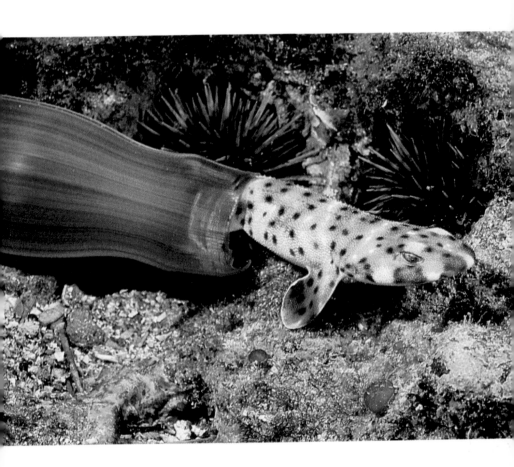

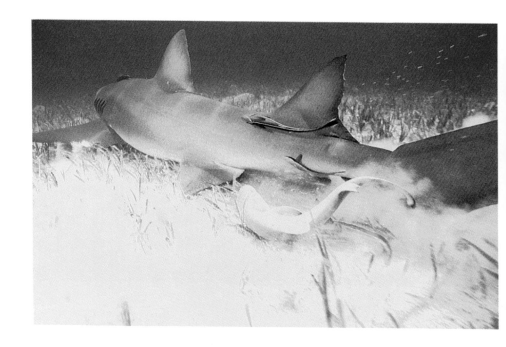

All pups grow from eggs.
In most sharks, the eggs grow inside
the mother.
They can grow there for nearly a year.

When ready, the pups come out of the
mother's body.
But they're not like human babies.
Pups take care of themselves from
the start.
Off they go, to begin the hunt for food.

CHAPTER FOUR

Fantastic Babies

Shark babies are called pups.
Shark mothers usually give birth to a
few pups at a time.

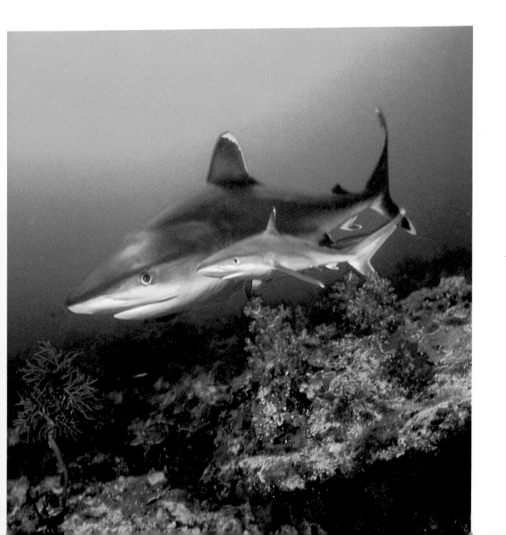

Swimming and breathing go together.
If sharks stop swimming, they stop breathing.
And they die.

Sharks breathe oxygen (say "OCK-suh-jun")
We breathe oxygen, too.
Our oxygen comes from the air.
Sharks get their oxygen from the water.

Most sharks swim with open mouths.
Water enters.
It flows over their gills.
The gills take the oxygen from the water.
Then the water flows out.

Swimming also keeps sharks afloat.
If they stop swimming, they sink to the bottom.

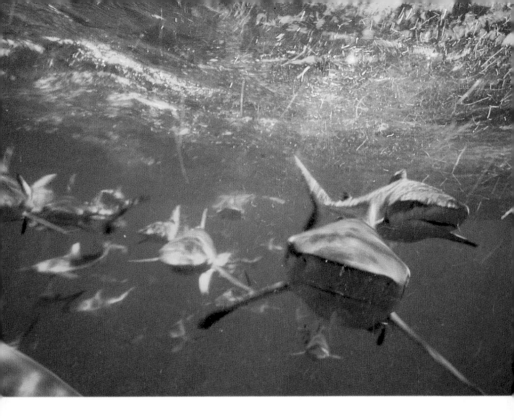

Sharks usually swim about three miles
per hour.
But they can put on bursts of speed.
When hunting, some reach 40 miles
per hour!

Did you know that most sharks swim
all the time?
They swim day and night.
They even swim when asleep!

Sharks do not have smooth scales like most fish.

Instead they have many sharp, pointed scales.

The points face back toward the tail.

They help water flow over the shark's body — without slowing it down.

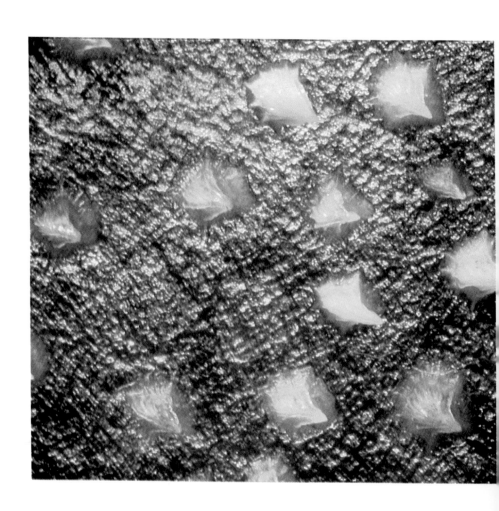

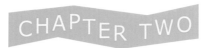

CHAPTER TWO

Powerful Swimmers

Sharks seem made for swimming.
Most have sleek, rounded bodies.
They slip easily through the water.

Sharks use their fins to swim.
The big tail fin swings from side to side.
The tail pushes against the water.
It moves the shark forward.
The other fins keep the shark steady
in the water.

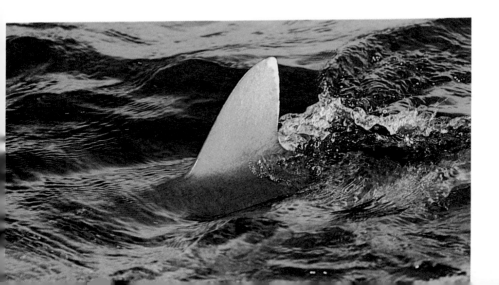

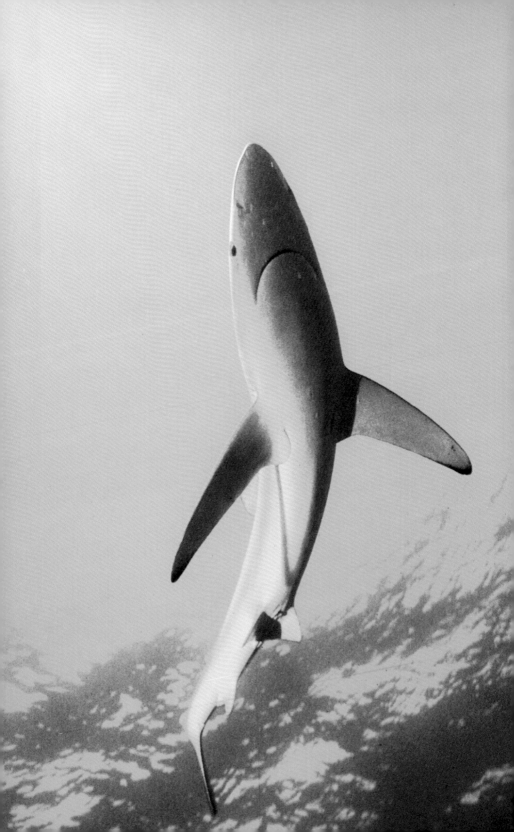

Most sharks hunt fish, seals, and porpoises.
But some eat dead or dying animals and shellfish.
A few kinds of sharks feed on tiny sea plants and animals.

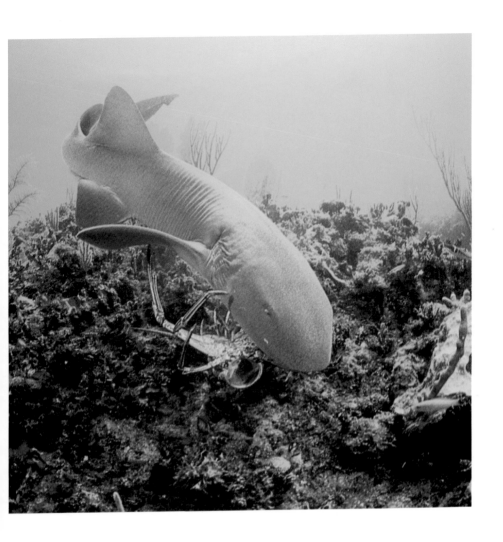

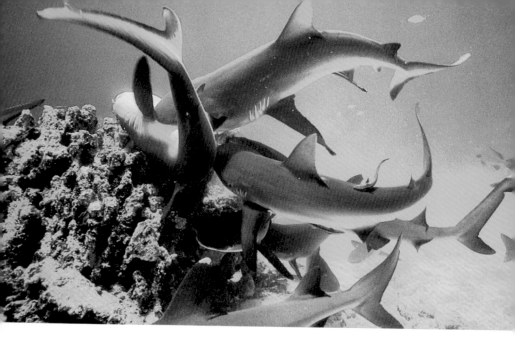

All at once, other sharks appear.
They churn and shake the water.
Each wants the same seal.

The sharks snap and rip at the seal.
They bite each other.
Sometimes they even bite themselves!
It's called a "feeding frenzy."

Soon there is little left of the seal.
The feeding frenzy is over.
The sharks glide away.

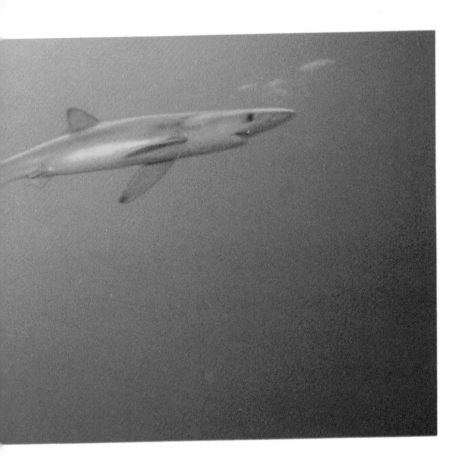

Suddenly the shark lunges.

CHOMP!

It sinks its teeth into the seal.

The shark rips off a large chunk
of flesh.

GULP!

The shark swallows it whole.

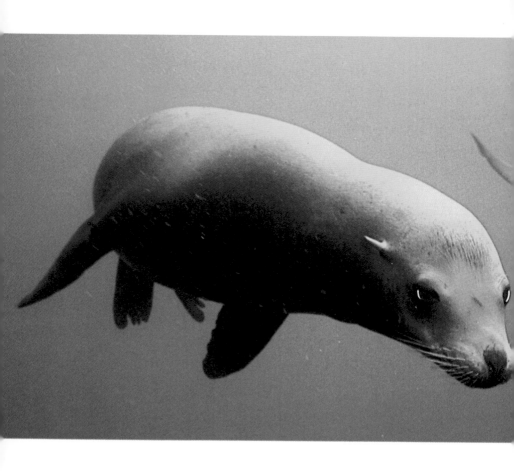

The water is dark.

But the shark sees well in little light.

It spots an injured seal.

The seal has been badly cut.

There is blood in the water.

The shark circles around.

It comes in closer and closer.

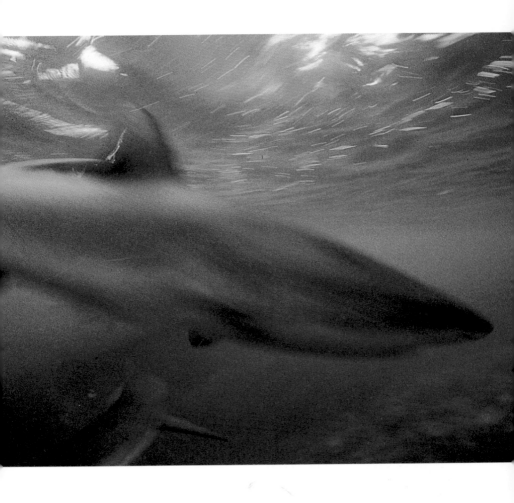

The shark also picks up some faraway
sounds.
The shark's ears are two small holes
in the skin.
It hears something moving in the water.
The shark swims even faster.

This hungry shark is swimming slowly back and forth.

Its senses are wide awake.

Suddenly the shark smells something.

It is blood in the water.

The blood is about a mile away.

That's as long as 20 blocks.

The shark speeds toward the smell.

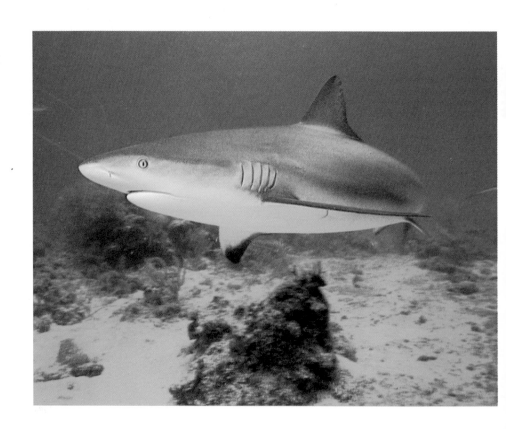

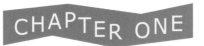

CHAPTER ONE

Great Hunters

Sharks are fish.

Most are very large.

They have huge appetites.

And they're almost always hunting for
something to eat.

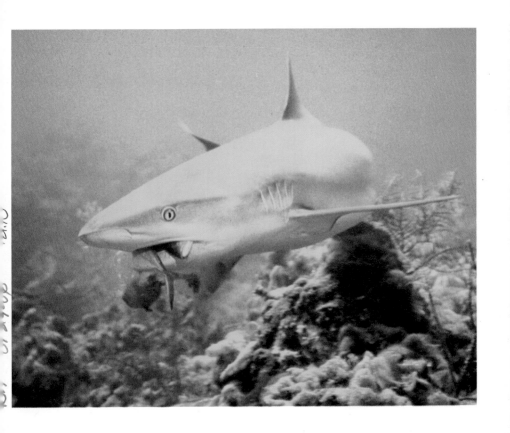

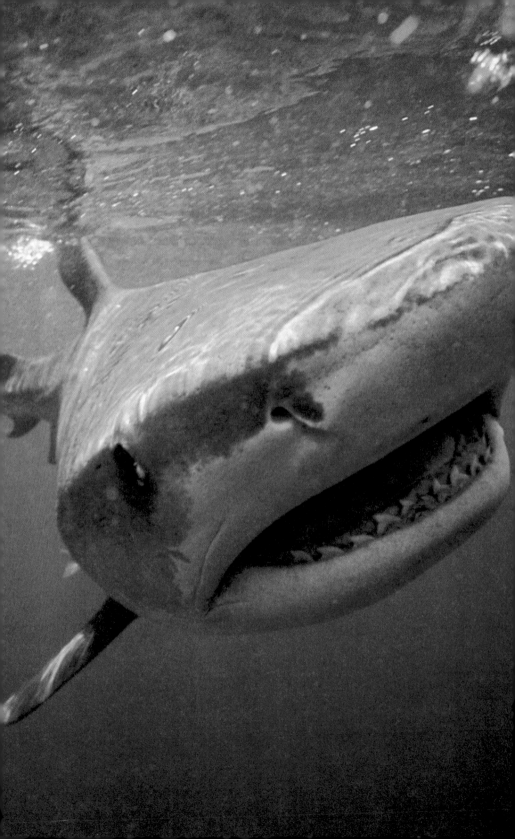

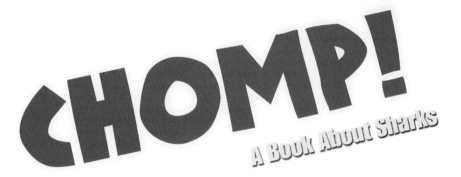

CHOMP!

A Book About Sharks

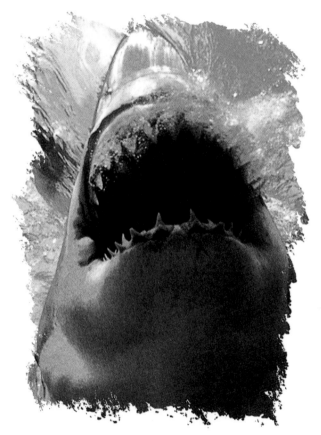

by Melvin Berger

Scholastic Reader — Level 3

Cartwheel BOOKS ®

SCHOLASTIC INC.

New York Toronto London Auckland Sydney
Mexico City New Delhi Hong Kong Buenos Aires

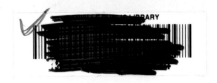

For the boys and girls
of the E.M. Baker School
— M.B.

Special thanks to Laurie Roulston
of the Denver Museum of Natural History
for her expertise

Photography credits:

Cover and page 3: James D. Watt/Innerspace Visions; pages 1 and 13: Bill Curtsinger; page 4: Ben Cropp/Innerspace Visions; page 5: Norbert Wu; page 6: Chris A. Crumley/EarthWater Stock Photography; page 7: Bill Curtsinger; pages 8-9: Mark Conlin/Innerspace Visions; page 10: Ron & Valerie Taylor/Innerspace Visions; page 11: Walt Stearns/Innerspace Visions; page 12: Norbert Wu/Peter Arnold, Inc.; page 14: Doug Perrine and Jose Castro/Innerspace Visions; page 15: Bill Curtsinger; page 17: Michael S. Nolan/Innerspace Visions; page 18: Michel Jozon/Innerspace Visions; page 19: Doug Perrine/Innerspace Visions; page 20: Mark Strickland/Innerspace Visions; pages 21-23: Jeff Rotman; page 24: Fred McConnaughey/Photo Researchers; page 25: Mark Strickland/Innerspace Visions; page 26: Doug Perrine/Innerspace Visions; page 27: Mark Conlin/Innerspace Visions; page 28: Massimo & Lucia Simion/Jeff Rotman; page 29: Jeff Rotman; page 30: Jeff Rotman/Innerspace Visions; page 31: David B. Fleetham/Innerspace Visions; page 32: Doug Perrine/Innerspace Visions; page 33: Bill Curtsinger; page 34: J. Dan Wright/EarthWater Stock Photography; page 35 top and bottom: Norbert Wu; page 36: Douglas Seifert/EarthWater Stock Photography; page 37: Bob Cranston/Innerspace Visions; page 38: Nigel Marsh/Innerspace Visions; page 39: Mark Conlin/Innerspace Visions; page 40: Kelvin Aitken/Peter Arnold, Inc.

Text copyright © 1999 by Melvin Berger.
Activities copyright © 2003 Scholastic Inc.

All rights reserved. Published by Scholastic Inc.
SCHOLASTIC, CARTWHEEL BOOKS, and associated logos are trademarks
and/or registered trademarks of Scholastic Inc.

Library of Congress Cataloging-in-Publication Data is available.

ISBN 0-590-52298-1

10 9 8 7 6 5 4   04 05 06 07
Printed in the U.S.A.   23
First printing, January 1999

Dear Parents,

Welcome to the Scholastic Reader series. We have taken over 80 years of experience with teachers, parents, and children and put it into a program that is designed to match your child's interests and skills.

Level 1—Short sentences and stories made up of words kids can sound out using their phonics skills and words that are important to remember.

Level 2—Longer sentences and stories with words kids need to know and new "big" words that they will want to know.

Level 3—From sentences to paragraphs to longer stories, these books have large "chunks" of texts and are made up of a rich vocabulary.

Level 4—First chapter books with more words and fewer pictures.

It is important that children learn to read well enough to succeed in school and beyond. Here are ideas for reading this book with your child:

- Look at the book together. Encourage your child to read the title and make a prediction about the story.
- Read the book together. Encourage your child to sound out words when appropriate. When your child struggles, you can help by providing the word.
- Encourage your child to retell the story. This is a great way to check for comprehension.
- Have your child take the fluency test on the last page to check progress.

Scholastic Readers are designed to support your child's efforts to learn how to read at every age and every stage. Enjoy helping your child learn to read and love to read.

—Francie Alexander
Chief Education Officer
Scholastic Education

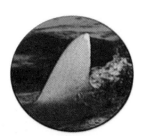